MEDICAL MYSTERIES

MEDICAL MYSTERIES

From the Bizarre to the Deadly...
The Cases That Have Baffled Doctors

Ann Reynolds AND
Kenneth Wapner

WITH CORINNE MOL

HYPERION

NEW YORK

Library of Congress Cataloging-in-Publication Data

Reynolds, Ann.
   Medical mysteries : from the bizarre to the deadly . . . the cases that have baffled doctors / Ann Reynolds and Kenneth Wapner ; with Corinne Mol.
       p.   cm.
   ISBN: 978-1-4013-0998-5 (alk. paper)
   1. Rare diseases—Popular works. I. Wapner, Kenneth. II. Mol, Corinne.
III. Title.
   RC48.8.R49 2009
   616—dc22
          2009018662

Book design by Karen Minster

FIRST EDITION

10   9   8   7   6   5   4   3   2   1

THIS BOOK IS DEDICATED,

WITH THANKS,

TO THE PATIENTS AND DOCTORS

WHO SHARED THEIR STORIES

WITH ABC NEWS

CONTENTS

MEDICAL MYSTERIES

INTRODUCTION

YOU SEE, I WAS SUPPOSED TO BE A DOCTOR.

Both my parents were physicians, and when I was little, most of the grown-ups I met had "Dr." in front of their names. I absorbed what seemed to be the obvious life lesson: when you grew up, you could be a doctor . . . or a patient. I knew which one to choose.

But somehow, in spite of being premed in college (yes, I even took Organic Chemistry), I ended up in television news. When ABC News decided to do a series on unusual medical conditions, it felt like redemption—another chance to dip my toe into medicine.

Remember the commercial that said, "I'm not a doctor, but I play one on TV"? That was the intriguing proposition that faced our producing team: without having to get medical degrees, we could try to understand some of the field's greatest puzzles. We could find people with unusual, extraordinary, bewildering medical conditions and tell their stories. And I was that most dangerous of creatures: a civilian with ten cents' worth of medical knowledge, mostly gleaned from my parents' dinner table conversations.

My mother was an anesthesiologist, so her hospital day

was done before my father's (internal medicine, specializing in liver disease). Dad would come home from the hospital as we set the table, take off his white medical coat and stethoscope, and we'd sit down to dinner. After a bit of family conversation, the daily game of "What's That Diagnosis?" would begin.

"We had a woman, sixty-three, admitted today with diffuse abdominal pain and delusions," Dad would offer.

"Something infectious, I think," my mom would reply, tossing the salad. "Any foreign travel? Did you test for parasites?"

They would bounce possible diagnoses back and forth, my mother always saying, "It's bound to be something more ordinary than *that*!" My father always held out for the rarer, more interesting condition.

My brother and I ate and occasionally contributed questions. (It's now very, very difficult to gross me out while I eat—I've heard it all.)

The process of narrowing down—taking the tiny clues from the patient's symptoms, genetics, the test results and scans, and finding out what was wrong and how to fix it—was something of a family sport. With the ABC News *Medical Mysteries* series, I got the chance to revisit the dinner table of my childhood and peek, once again, into the way doctors think and diseases work.

THE SHOW STRUCK A CHORD with television audiences, I think, because we all live in bodies—we're all wondering if that little ache or that strange sound in our neck could "be something." Perhaps, if you're not in the medical field, some of the syndromes and conditions in this book will seem, well, impossible. Who would guess there could be seizures set off by music alone? Who would think that people who seem completely normal, who have entirely normal vision, might be simply unable to "see" human faces? Did you know that some people are born with their internal organs backwards inside them? Or that a particular form of paralysis strikes only first-time surfers? And another can be set off by eating a pizza? And what kind of medical problem would make a man look as though he was turning into a tree, with "roots" and "bark"?

We're the ones who got to find out and tell you about these incredible things. But as fascinated as we all were by the exotic conditions and inventive medical treatments, the more stories we looked into, the more we realized: these stories were powerful because they happened to *people*. Normal, ordinary people who live through symptoms they've never expected—and normal, ordinary doctors who painstakingly unravel diseases and struggle to give their patients relief and, perhaps, even cure them.

All the patients and doctors involved in *Medical Mysteries* were kind enough to let us into their worlds and take us on their journeys. Most of them did it so that people out there with the same set of problems will know that there's a diagnosis and, often, treatment available to them. It was a privilege to put their experiences in front of the public.

As you read through the book, as you picture all the scans, all the tests, all the questions, all the symptoms—you may end up like our team at ABC News did: just flat-out amazed. With billions of cells and processes and checks and balances inside our bodies—systems we ignore as we read the paper and go to work and drop the kids off at a playdate—be amazed that it doesn't go wrong more often. Be amazed at how lucky most of are every day—every healthy day.

—Ann Reynolds

1. THE TREE MAN

MEDICAL MYSTERIES ARE FASCINATING SCIENTIFIC PUZZLES— you watch some of the smartest, most intuitive people on Earth, in world renowned medical centers, track down the tiny genetic problem or microbe that has wreaked havoc in a human body.

And then there are others that tug at you further—like the story of the "tree man."

It sounded almost like a fable when we first heard of it: a man in a remote area of Indonesia who seemed to be turning into a tree. Over the course of many years, his face, body, and especially his hands and feet, seemed to become more and more covered with what looked like bark and roots. Was it a medical condition, an exotic syndrome that no one had ever heard of? Was he even real?

ABC News has a reporter based in Jakarta, Margaret Conley, and we asked her to investigate. She set off into the heart of Indonesia. Her report? It was all true, and it became one of the most fascinating cases we'd ever covered, and one that spoke not only to our curiosity about Dede Koswara's medical issues, but to what it means to be able to see past surface appearance to the human being underneath.

A SIMPLE WART?

Dede grew up in a remote village in Indonesia, a three-hour drive and two boat rides from Jakarta. His home is as green and lush as you can imagine—fields planted with crops, sleepy dirt roads, palm trees, and flowering vines. His family fished for most of their food and lived a simple village life—no running water or telephones. His mother's name is Engkar (we discovered that in Indonesia, almost everyone is known simply by one name). She says that when he was young, Dede was exactly the same as the other boys in the village, riding his bike and playing soccer with his friends.

Then a simple wart on Dede's teenaged knee seemed to become infected—the family didn't understand why the problem wouldn't go away. He developed additional warts on his face and hands.

"The children teased me," says Dede. "But my family protected me."

As is custom in Dede's village, he married young, before he was twenty.

"When Dede was getting married, he was a normal guy with normal hands and feet," says his father, Ateng. He could do anything with his hands, they told us, and worked building and repairing houses, providing for a growing family. It was after the birth of his first child, a son, Entis, that the warts started to spread; after the birth of his second child, a daughter, Entang, they grew all over his body, and the warts on his hands increased in size.

Dede and his family are Muslim—at the mosque they prayed for him to get better. But Dede's condition only

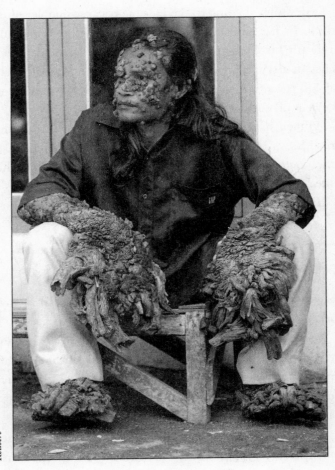

Reuters

worsened. His legs, face, arms, chest, and especially his hands and feet became covered with growths. On his hands and feet, they grew into what looked like roots—long, curving spurs six or seven inches long. He began to look like the trees surrounding his house.

Dede stopped going to the mosque because people stared at him. In fact, he stopped going out altogether. He could barely lift his hands or feet, which were now about fifteen inches in circumference. He couldn't feed or dress himself, and his parents took him to a local doctor for treatment. They cut off some warts—to no avail.

"Fifteen days after the operation, they grew back and spread," says Dede's father. The next bit of medical advice? "The doctor offered the solution—to cut [off] both of his hands," says Dede's mother. "I was so sad."

His parents decided to take Dede home—no amputations.

A PERFECT STORM

His wife asked for a divorce because Dede couldn't work anymore.

"I accepted the decision," his father says. "We weren't angry. As a parent, because I love my son, I said okay, if he wants to move in with us, that's our duty as parents. He came to live at our house." The children went to live with Dede's sister-in-law.

Dede stayed cloistered in his parents' home. His sister went to work to support them. His mother made special shirts for him with ties at the side seams, because his hands, covered with "roots," couldn't fit through a normal sleeve. "I didn't go anywhere. I stayed at home," says Dede.

Desperate to bring some money to the family, he did the only thing he could think of to survive: he went to a nearby city, Bandung, and begged on the streets.

What happened next, what most people would recoil at, would end up being the key to his medical treatment. Because Dede was about to become famous.

Hanny Enterprises runs a profitable freak show. For 10,000 rupiah (about a dollar), the public sees feats of strength, strange exhibitions of unusual abilities (one performer can eat glass), and gets a look at people whose appearance is outside the ordinary.

Hanny made "Tree Man" a star. "I didn't make any promises," says Hanny. "Rather than [having] him stay home, not doing anything and being a burden to his family, it means that if he joins, lots of people will come and show pity on him and help him."

People flocked to Hanny's show, and doctors were as interested in Dede as the rest of the public. They decided to find out what on earth was going on in his body. It turned out to be a "perfect storm" of dermatology: perhaps the worst case of warts (usually considered just a minor annoyance) known to medical science today, coupled with an unusual inability to fight them off. A common virus (one you've got if you've ever had a wart!) was taking over Dede's skin.

"This is the most remarkable case, the most severe case, I have seen in my career," says Dr. Anthony Gaspari from the University of Maryland, who specializes in immune function of the skin. "I was actually asked by the Discovery Channel to join them and to study this patient and confirm what kind of health problem he had."

SO WHAT IS A WART?

A small medical digression: what are warts, anyway?

"Warts are viral growths on the skin, creating extensions of the skin, which have a full blood supply—they become part of the skin," says New York City dermatologist Dr. Debra Jaliman, an assistant professor of Dermatology at Mt. Sinai School of Medicine. "They can occur anywhere. Warts are caused by the human papilloma virus (HPV) and are very common. Anybody can get warts."

Jaliman says warts are very contagious and kids get them from playing with other kids. "They touch other kids' hands that have warts," says Jaliman. "Sometimes the children take baths with their siblings, so all the kids in the family get warts. You can get it from the surface of a public pool. They are very common, and if you don't treat them, they can stay within the skin's surface. If you have it on one finger, it can go to the finger adjacent to it. And sometimes people think that if they have one wart it's going to go away, and they don't treat it. Then they have ten warts and twenty warts and sometimes we see one hundred warts. So it can become a big problem."

Jaliman cautions that warts need to be treated, and over-the-counter remedies can work. But, if the problem persists, a dermatologist should be consulted. She treats patients with liquid nitrogen, which freezes the warts, and sometimes prescribes stronger acids that you can get at a pharmacy to burn away the growths. Other medicines? Immune stimulators (creams that stimulate the body's immune system to destroy the wart virus) and even, in the worst cases, laser treatment.

The treatments don't leave scars; they're straightforward and relatively easy to do, but, says Jaliman, "You have to be persistent and very aggressive. Some people don't do well with the treatments because their immune system isn't that good at fighting the virus. It's always better to treat a virus early. In other words, if you get one wart, it's a lot easier to treat than if you have twenty warts. So I always encourage parents—if you start to see warts on your kids, come early and get the virus treated."

DEDE'S CASE

Dede, clearly, didn't get those early treatments, and with his unique immune system problem, they may not have worked. "I've never seen a case that extreme," Jaliman says of Dede. "If he was treated early and he was treated aggressively, I think he might have had a better outcome. But, you know, it's always so unfair to say because we aren't there, and we didn't treat him."

Jaliman agrees with medical experts who have written about Dede—it's clear there was something wrong with his immune system.

"When I think back to the early days of AIDS," she says, "the patients I saw before we had medication for AIDS, their warts looked like that. They were warts that just grew totally out of control. And it was so difficult to treat because the body has *some* defense against the wart virus. When you see *no* defense and the virus growing totally out of control, it takes over the skin. The skin looks almost totally unrecognizable. That's when you know there is something wrong with the immune system."

In Indonesia, Dede is now under the care of a team of local doctors at Hasan Sadikin Hospital. Dr. Hardisiswo Soedjana, who is known as Dr. Hardi, is the lead doctor in Dede's case.

"When Dede came here, I saw almost all of the body of Dede had warts," says Hardi. "As long as the virus is still in his body, there can be growths."

Gaspari, with his specialty in immune function of the skin, has been in contact with the Indonesian doctors and has visited Indonesia twice to help treat Dede.

"We've learned that Dede has a defect in his immune system that doesn't allow him to control this viral infection," says Gaspari. "One of our approaches will be to help restore his immune system. Secondly, we will be attacking the virus to cause the regression of these tumorous growths on his skin. We are trying to obtain some of the pharmaceutical agents that we need to give this treatment, and to deal with some of the complications that we've noted. We're planning further studies to understand the disease. So everything that he needs will be provided to him here in Indonesia. It would be very disruptive for him to travel to the United States. He's much more comfortable here close to his home and his family."

A team of doctors at Hasan Sadikin Hospital has performed eight surgeries over nine months. While Dede was under anesthesia, doctors had to improvise a bit: they'd never done surgery like this before.

"We estimated that the time of one surgery would be just two hours, but it was prolonged to four hours," says Hardi.

Doctors ended up using a small electric saw to cut off the longest wart growths—dead skin tissue hardened by the years. In just one surgery, they filled surgical pans with pounds of what had looked like Dede's "roots" from his hands and feet.

"The stuff that you see in the bowl that the doctors cut off from Dede, that's actually the wart virus," Jaliman said when we showed her a still photo taken from the hospital videotape recording of the operation. "That is a pile of contagious viral skin. I think it's such a tragic thing for somebody to have to live with something like this," she adds. "Imagine when people look at him and they see that, they have no idea what it is. It's terrible for him because it is, in fact, contagious. So imagine what his life must be like. People don't want to go near him."

Doctors are hopeful that Dede's quality of life can improve, most of all that he will be able to use his hands again. The medical team wants to use skin grafts to replace areas of skin that have been severely damaged by the wart growths. They'll be "harvesting" some undamaged skin from near his stomach. However, Gaspari cautions, there is a limit to what can be done.

"The most important part [of the surgeries] is to restore the function of his hands and feet," Hardi says. "He was given a tissue expander to grow more skin on his abdomen. I have explained to him and his family that it's unlikely that he's ever going to be completely cured of his condition. He has an internal health problem that is allowing this to happen, and he's going to be living with that health problem for the remainder of his life." Hardi adds that it will be a challenge to keep Dede in an improved state.

A GENTLE MAN

If all this is giving you the creeps, we can't offer much solace. Dr. Jaliman says the HPV virus is everywhere—there's a reason they call it the "common" wart.

"If you have a micro-abrasion in your skin, which we all have, if you have a paper cut or you have *anything*, and there is a virus, it's going to go into your skin, and you're going to get it," Jaliman says. "Anybody can get a virus and that's why it spreads so easily, and that's why I treat so many warts in my practice."

Fortunately, Dede's condition does not seem to be hereditary, so his children and grandchildren don't appear to have inherited his illness. His children have loved him throughout, no matter what he's looked like.

At the end of the day, what struck us most was the gentle, accepting man behind the story. Decades of difficulty don't seem to have made him bitter. We interviewed Dede after the first of the series of surgeries—which took away most of the "bark" and returned his feet and hands to a more human shape. He said his hands feel lighter, he can hold things with his thumb, and we watched as, with glee, he completed a crossword puzzle. He delights in the hope of an ordinary life. "I want to find a job, be able to hang out with friends," he says.

His parents say Dede has always left his fate to Allah. "I have accepted the condition and have asked God to give me strength," Dede says. "My spirit is lifted because of this operation. I'm very happy. I got my spirit back."

2. PERSISTENT SEXUAL AROUSAL SYNDROME

I KNOW, I KNOW. YOU PROBABLY GIGGLED WHEN YOU READ THE title of this chapter. And thought, "Hmmm, too much of a good thing!" The problem is, the women who suffer from this syndrome—and they do suffer—have heard it all before. And they are not amused.

Turns out wall-to-wall orgasms, all day every day, are no fun at all. And if you're a little startled by the frank speech of the women who have persistent sexual arousal syndrome, remember: for some of them, this is a daily—hourly—concern, and they are grateful to have a chance to talk about it at all.

In 1995, when Heather Dearmon was in her late twenties and began to feel as though she was constantly on the edge of orgasm, she thought it was because she was pregnant and her fetus was somehow putting pressure on her pelvis. But after she gave birth, the sensation only intensified, and she found only one way to stop it.

"I would be masturbating morning, afternoon, and night," Heather says. "When you're masturbating so much—I had to buy a vibrator because you get tired. Most of my time was spent doing that. So I put my son (he was two at the time) in day care. And I would be crying while I was masturbating, because, I mean, nobody wants to do that all day long."

Heather and her husband, Jeremy, are now in their thirties. He sells guitars online from their home in suburban Columbia, South Carolina. They've been dealing with PSAS for just about their entire fourteen-year marriage. It's rare, and doctors can barely diagnose it, much less cure it. In many marriages, men wish their spouse had more sexual desire; for the Dearmons, Heather's perpetual arousal is torture.

A VERY PRIVATE HELL

"I have considered surgery just to cut everything off 'down there,'" Heather comments. "I would rather never have another orgasm for the rest of my life."

Jeremy says that while Heather is the one at the mercy of her body, they are in this together. "The women are the ones who are suffering. But it's definitely mutual in a marriage. Both lives are affected by it. It's not a personal decision that the woman has made."

This condition wasn't even *diagnosable* until a few years ago. We were worried that we wouldn't be able to find women comfortable talking about it. We'd forgotten something pretty basic to human nature: when you're suffering, one way to feel better is to feel that you're helping someone else. Each of the women we talked to had lived in a very private hell, thinking this syndrome was somehow her "fault." Each of them wanted to let others know that it's a medical problem—that if there isn't an immediate cure, there's at least a community. We asked doctors who treat PSAS to talk to their patients and ask: is there any chance you'd want to tell a television audience what you're going through? Some were comfortable using their whole names; some only wanted to be known by their first names. We thought the topic was important, and if they were brave enough to talk about it, we would be happy to use whatever names they gave us.

Dr. Irwin Goldstein, clinical professor of Surgery at University of California at San Diego and head of Sexual Medicine at Alvarado Hospital, is one of the few researchers studying persistent sexual arousal syndrome (PSAS).

"Every lecture I give on this, there's always smirks in the audience," he says. " 'Oh, I wish my wife was like this.' These are professional physicians."

Goldstein is unequivocal: "You do not want your wife to have this. The genitals are aroused twenty-four seven, three hundred and sixty-five days a year."

Women who have PSAS, he says, can't concentrate or work. Anything that moves or vibrates will lead them into orgasmic release. The process of orgasm will tend to temporarily rid them of their engorgement. However, the state of being "on the brink" soon returns.

"Ice is very common," says Goldstein. "We have a woman who ices a condom and puts the condom in the genitalia to basically survive the day."

It's important that you understand: PSAS should not be confused with what people typically think of as nymphomania— an uncontrollable and insatiable desire for sex. Goldstein says that sex is the *last* thing that is usually on the minds of women with PSAS: "They are totally focused on their genitalia. They have no interest in sex, their body is playing a trick on them. They can't be productive. They don't know where to go for help. [They] are even afraid to tell people that they have PSAS for fear that they'll think they're perverts."

All types of women are afflicted. "We have professional teachers," says Goldstein. "If these women announced that's what they had, other teachers, or parents, wouldn't want their daughters and sons to be taught by a sexual 'deviant.' We have professional physicians, attorneys. We have artists, writers, and moms. I would venture to say that around the world there are thousands of women with PSAS."

Most doctors have never heard of PSAS, which was only isolated as a medical condition in 2001. Before that, doctors and patients had no way to define it. Goldstein now classifies it as "spontaneous, intrusive, and unwanted genital arousal, consisting of throbbing, pulsing, or tingling without the person's sexual interest or desire."

Goldstein says that one of the most difficult aspects of the condition is that most women suffer alone—or think that they are the only ones in the world with persistent, involuntary orgasm.

"How would you like to be in a situation where you had absolutely no control of the reflex?" Goldstein says. "It activated whenever it wanted, wherever it wanted, and you were walking around in a situation with engorged genitalia on the verge of having an orgasm in the middle of a place that was absolutely not private? Most women who have PSAS don't even know they have it. Or that there's help for them."

Goldstein likens the sexual reflex to the bladder reflex. Babies have an uninhibited bladder reflex and wear diapers. As they grow into young children, they learn to control that reflex. We come to understand that it's socially inappropriate, and messy, to wet one's pants. It's the same, Goldstein says, with sex: "When you're interested in sex, when you're in the appropriate intimate situation, and the time is correct and you're with the right person, you activate the reflex."

Heather says that Goldstein's bladder analogy is apt: "It's like having a really, really full bladder. And you know the way you think about, when you have a really full bladder, you just want to be able to go to the bathroom and have relief. You just want some peace in your body."

Heather kept trying to tame what she called her "beast." She says it completely disrupted her life, her social relationships, and her sense of herself. She tried to focus on other things aside from her genitals but found that impossible. She stopped going to church, shopping for food, traveling.

"I just couldn't do anything," she says. "There was one time for me where it was really unbelievably bad and we were on a really long trip with family. And I actually went into a public restroom and masturbated to make it go away. It was absolutely humiliating and degrading."

She decided there was only one way out. "I knew I was going to commit suicide," she says. "I mean, it was that bad." When she saw that her thoughts were taking that route, Heather became so frightened that she would lose her mind or take her own life that she committed herself to a psychiatric hospital.

Her humiliation and despair were complete when, in the hospital, surrounded by medical professionals who were supposed to be trying to help her, Heather says, "the nurse came in and said, 'Honey, I wish I could stay home and masturbate all day long.' I also had one doctor suggest I become a lesbian."

"I'M NOT ALONE"

It was by a stroke of luck that one day Jeremy discovered a magazine article that described his wife's symptoms exactly. Jeremy quickly showed it to Heather: "She immediately started crying and [said]: 'Oh, my God, I'm not alone!'"

Heather had found the upside: other women had PSAS. The downside? There is no cure for the condition. Goldstein and others in the field say it can be treated, however. They've experimented with treating PSAS with antidepressants. Heather takes Paxil now to "reset" her sexual reflex. And while it doesn't work for everyone, the drug has reduced her symptoms to a more manageable level.

Any hormonal change can trigger PSAS—menopause or, in Heather's case, pregnancy. In some cases, Goldstein has even treated menopausal women for PSAS that began when they simply changed their hormonal therapy. But ironically, it is sometimes the very type of drugs that Heather is now taking to *treat* her symptoms—antidepressants—that *triggers* PSAS in others.

Although PSAS occurs in the genitals, doctors say that it is regulated by the central nervous system. "Clearly, drugs or events such as pregnancy and menopause affect the central nervous system," says Goldstein. "Millions of women take antidepressants, and one of the largest side effects is sexual disorders. We recognize that inhibitory neurotransmitters, such as serotonin and the classic antidepressant agents, inhibit sexual response. And we recognize that dopamine is an excitatory neurotransmitter, and agents that increase dopamine can increase sexual function. Parkinson's patients who take dopamine will have improved interest and orgasmic potential. So we understand that."

That is about as much as researchers using antidepressants to treat PSAS *do* know, Goldstein cautions. He says that the repeated and constant need to orgasm could be "visualized" as a form of recurrent seizure activity that activates in an area of the brain without volition. His patients' MRIs and CAT scans, however, have revealed nothing. Goldstein adds that there has been one link established in the medical literature: women who *stop* taking antidepressant medications sometimes begin PSAS. Indeed, a paper published in the *Journal of Sexual Medicine* reports that a woman polled members of her support group for PSAS—60 or 70 percent believed that their PSAS began with sudden discontinuation of antidepressants.

WHEN YOU CAN'T EVEN UNDERSTAND what causes a syndrome, a cure is elusive. "I don't think pharmacologic management is going to be the long-term answer," says Goldstein. "I think especially those who have virtually no inhibition of this reflex live a complicated life and are the worst off."

Goldstein says the link between the inability to fully empty the bladder and PSAS may help doctors treat the disorder. "One of the things women patients don't tell us, but that we get out of doing a detailed history, is when their genitals are engorged, it's difficult to urinate," Goldstein notes. "They never empty their bladder; they hardly ever go to the bathroom. When they do urinate, instead of it being a full stream, it's short and staccato. That's because their tissues are engorged. Their pelvic floor is contracting. One idea is to take women who have the voiding dysfunction and see what effect pelvic neuromodulation has on their PSAS."

What is pelvic neuromodulation? Patients lie flat on an examination table. A pillow is placed under the pelvis; the lower back is anesthetized, and a needle and a wire are put directly into the opening in the spinal cord where the nerve root S3 comes out. Electricity runs into the wire to stimulate the nerve. Goldstein says women with overactive bladder function who undergo the procedure say, "Wow, I don't have to go to the bathroom anymore." He says that the hope is that when they have the wire fired for them, women with PSAS will have a similar response. The engorgement in their genitals will decrease, and they will once again be in control over their state of sexual arousal.

That is, as much as any woman (or man) is ever in control. After all, the relationship of the physical and the emotional, that combination we call female "desire," is something doctors have never been able to quantify. How much of a woman's sexual arousal is hardwired in the brain, in other words is physical, and how much depends on the relationship, the emotions involved? Physicians would love to know, especially after 1999's bombshell report in the *Journal of the American Medical Association* indicated that 43 percent of American women experienced sexual dysfunction. The push to study it (to test Viagra in women, to test hormone creams) hasn't yet revealed what doctors can *do* about it.

BACK TO PSAS and the attempted treatment of this very physical problem—it seems that neuromodulation sometimes has no effect. Nancy Austin tried it. "I saw a local vaginal specialist," says Nancy. "And he's the one who told me it was the pudendal nerve which was being overstimulated. So I had three pudendal nerve blocks, which are extremely painful, and they didn't even work."

Still, Goldstein says, he thinks the key to controlling the disorder may be neurological treatment—with the addition of a therapy that fell into disrepute in decades past: electroconvulsive therapy. Doctors throw a surge of electrical energy through the brain and nervous system, causing a seizure, hoping to "reset" the brain at normal levels. It was called "shock therapy" or "electroshock" in the 1940s and '50s, and seen as a cure for just about any desperate psychological condition, from bipolar disorder to schizophrenia. Later it was widely discredited and pretty much discarded as a treatment option. In the past decade or so, however, doctors have tried it again in limited cases, and found it actually has medical benefits for some with clinical depression.

"We have a woman who was suicidal and very depressed and, just for the indications of suicide and depression, underwent electroconvulsive therapy," Goldstein says. "She had PSAS, and miraculously she emailed me that her PSAS was under control after the electroconvulsive therapy. We don't recommend that people go to that extreme, but it was evidence to me that by her resolving her PSAS with a neurological treatment—electroconvulsive therapy—we were able to control this horrible syndrome." He notes that therapy, to remain effective, has to be repeated on a regular basis.

Some women find that doing exercises like the Kegel—in which they squeeze the pubococcygeal and the vaginal muscles—provides relief.

There are different types of PSAS. Emily, another woman suffering from PSAS, told us that masturbation doesn't really alleviate the discomfort of the syndrome. "For me, stimulation, none of that would work for me, because [my condition] is more internal. I need to do the Kegel," the exercises familiar to postpartum women—they're often used to increase bladder control.

"I need something to get it from a different angle: an internal way of working and massaging," Emily adds.

Women with PSAS often have trouble sleeping. Heather says she was often up, masturbating in the middle of the night. "I'd be asleep for a couple of hours and then [the sensations] would wake me up. And I would have to masturbate all over again," she says.

Lauren, another woman with PSAS, says: "I don't sleep for days sometimes, maybe an hour at about five in the morning. There [have] been nights when I'm walking, pacing in my bedroom when it's really strong, and I just want to die. I just want it to stop."

"Normal people often have sex just before going to sleep and it relaxes them," says Goldstein. "While sleeping, their genitals are inhibited, they have the baseline flaccid state of genital arousal. Can you imagine how difficult going to sleep would be if you constantly had an erection or your clitoris or labia were constantly engorged to the point where it's just ready to undergo orgasmic relief?"

HOW ABOUT MEN?

This is primarily a female condition, but Goldstein estimates that there are also thousands of men who have a similar syndrome—no control over their erections. "We've done a little more research on the men [because] we have a longer history of treatment with men who have sexual problems," says Goldstein. "Idiopathic recurrent prolonged penile erection would be the equivalent of persistent sexual arousal."

That's a little different from something called priapism, named after the Greek god of Eros, Priapus. Priapism is unwanted and prolonged engorgement of the penis that lasts for more than four hours, and it's considered a medical emergency because blood can't circulate back into the body. The complications can include blood clots and gangrene.

The treatment for these male disorders is unpleasant, to say the least—a syringe loaded with insulin injected into the penis to release adrenaline. The adrenaline significantly contracts the muscles of the penis and the erection goes down. "It's not that much fun to stick a needle in your penis every day to make it go down so you can go to work," Goldstein notes, adding that it's often difficult for people with sexual problems to get the help they need, even today when Viagra has become a household word and is used by millions.

The ideal way to work with PSAS is a coordinated multidisciplinary therapy, says Goldstein, and you have to treat somebody else in addition to the sufferer. "We would also work with the partner, we would work with *their* anxiety and stress and depression."

This, of course, is the ideal. The public spotlight on Viagra and erectile dysfunction notwithstanding, the sexual problems of women (and many of the lesser known problems of men, for that matter) are looked at askance, perhaps even ridiculed. Women who seek help for PSAS usually have a very different experience than the multi-pronged approach Goldstein outlines above.

"One woman described to me being in the doctor's office, telling the nurse practitioner who comes in first what her problem was," says Goldstein. "The nurse practitioner goes outside—she hears laughter. Men who have erection problems are laughed at. We have HIV medicine, sleep medicine, pain medicine, and family medicine. It would be good to have sexual medicine as a specialty. Someone who has a sexual problem should find a health-care provider and a facility that has multidisciplines to take care of people who have sexual problems. There wouldn't be any laughter under such circumstances. It's my dream to see that this comes to fruition, but we're just not there yet."

IT'S WHAT WE CHOOSE

In today's world, people struggling with PSAS do the best they can. Heather and Jeremy remain committed in their marriage through the trials and tribulations of PSAS.

"It's not like he couldn't satisfy me sexually," says Heather. "It has nothing to do with him. There is just something going on in my body that I have no control over. He helped me by staying away from me. He helped me by learning rejection. That hurt both of us—but I didn't even want him touching me."

"We can only be affectionate at certain times," says Jeremy. "I need to take that easy."

"Sometimes I have to stop him from kissing me," says Heather with regret. "Still, I believe we're honestly, happily married. It's what we still choose. We love one another."

3. A BAD SMELL

ANOTHER STRANGE SYNDROME. ANOTHER UNPRONOUNCEABLE name. Except this time we are talking about the rarest of the rare—a disorder with only six hundred cases diagnosed worldwide.

You've heard the phrase "something smells fishy." But for the brave and beautiful women you're about to meet, that smell is the story of their lives.

Camille, who, for reasons of privacy, only wants to be known by her first name, is somebody who has "got it all." Looks: she's a former model. Brains: she has an honors degree, a master's in teaching. But she has something else as well: trimethylaminuria (TMAU for short), a genetic metabolic disorder which causes about 10 percent of those who have it to reek of spoiled fish.

When one of our medical producers raised "fish odor syndrome" in a meeting—that's one of its medical nicknames—there was a moment of stunned silence.

"You mean that's a real syndrome?"

"You mean they just smell like fish?"

"Can't they just wash it off?"

"You're kidding, right?"

"Is it permanent?"

"What on earth could cause it?"

When producers who are sorting through every manner of strange disorder ask *that* many questions, you know it's a condition that everyone else will be just as curious about.

A DEEP DARK ODOR

Camille is gorgeous—honey-blond wavy hair, a delicate face, tall, and slender. And yet, without being able to help it, she emits the pungent, unpleasant odor of rotting fish. It doesn't matter how many times a day she showers or what kind of soap or deodorant she uses. She loves teaching, but says her students didn't want to come near her; they said that her classroom stank of dead fish. They even made up a nickname for her: "Miss Fishy."

For most of her life, the odor coming from her body was a complete mystery to Camille. "I didn't know why I was emitting such a strong odor," Camille says. "And it's not just body odor. It can fill an entire room. And recently, it filled an auditorium."

An auditorium? That's right.

"It's a very heavy, intense, dark, deep smell," she says.

Her job as a teacher became excruciating.

"I would open windows," she says. "I would leave the door open. I would put fans in my classrooms. I mean, the whole nine yards. I was so focused on—Do I smell? Are they saying things? Are they whispering? Are they laughing? I would cry all the way home from school. All the time. Same thing that I used to go through for my whole life."

A TRAIL OF TEARS

Since Camille was a little girl, the smell that seeps from her pores (and is, in a cruel twist of fate, also carried by her tears) has made Camille's life miserable. Her ordeal began in first grade.

"One of my teachers asked me if I was showering every day. And from that point on, she kind of sat me in the corner of the classroom. And kids would call me a freak. They would tell me I smelled like horse manure. Dead fish."

For a little girl, that kind of ostracism was almost too much to bear. We're instinctively programmed to stay away from smells like dead fish because that helps keep us from eating spoiled or dangerous food—and the other children stayed away from her.

It has been both a blessing and a curse that Camille couldn't detect the smell on herself, which is part of the syndrome. The odor's intensity fluctuates from day to day, and she never knows when it is out of control.

Her condition led to frequent humiliation. Her aborted first kiss in sixth grade set a precedent for the future.

"I was with a bunch of friends," she recalls. "We used to go to this cemetery. Everyone would pair off in couples to kiss. The boy that I was with refused to get close to me and refused to kiss me. I couldn't quite understand it. The next day I went to school, and someone had taped a note on my locker that said: 'You need to take a shower. You need to brush your teeth.' He told everyone in school that I was an unclean person and my breath smelled like horse manure, and I smelled like dead fish. I had an incident in middle school where a bunch of kids cornered me in the cafeteria and threw tuna fish sandwiches at me. I became very isolated. And still to this day, I tend to be socially reclusive. When someone tells you you're a freak, you're dirty, you're disgusting, you start to believe it. When you're told that in very crucial development stages, you think it must be true. I had a sibling who would tell me no one is ever going to love you because you stink. I always thought: 'I'm a freak. If you only knew the truth about me—my dirty little secret.' And you start to see yourself as 'other.' Not quite human, not quite animal either. Just some kind of *other*."

Camille says that in high school she dated a guy who repeatedly told her that she smelled of dead fish. "Sometimes it was said to me in the heat of passion, and very cruelly," says Camille. "And, of course, that had a serious effect because I trusted and loved this person."

In her adult life, Camille has had a serious relationship with someone who had a deviated septum. "He had no sense of smell whatsoever," she says. "So that worked to my benefit."

The last long-term relationship she was in felt like a minefield. Camille was constantly jumping through hoops, living in a state of apprehension of being found out and rejected. She led what amounted to a secret life behind her boyfriend's back, always on edge, afraid of being "outed."

"I got very good about spraying myself with all kinds of things," Camille says. "He would come over to my house unannounced. If I hadn't gone through my little ritual of spraying myself, I wouldn't open the door. I would just avoid him. I was constantly breaking our plans if I had any remote suspicion that I was having an odor problem. I loved this person. I wanted this person to respect me. I didn't want to be ridiculed and shamed. So I never said anything to him. . . . He did say that sometimes my breath would smell—badly. That's one of the ways that the odor comes out. Sometimes I just wouldn't get too close to him, or be intimate with him, because I was panicked."

It wasn't just her social life that was difficult. Work was problematic. One of her first jobs was as a teller in a credit union. Her supervisor sprayed her work area with perfume and Lysol. She was eventually put in the drive-through section of the bank, away from the other employees and separated from customers.

Camille went to doctor after doctor, internists, and gynecologists. No one helped. No one could tell her what was wrong. A chiropractor she went to for an unrelated back problem told her that she needed to "detox." She felt helpless and hopeless—and even considered taking her own life. And just months after she started that dream teaching job, her first with her new master's degree, Camille quit under the strain.

In a deep depression, Camille was on the Internet when a lucky click brought her the answer to the mysterious problem that had plagued her for as long as she could remember. She typed in "fishy body odor" and TMAU came up on the screen. With increasing disbelief, she learned that the condition was caused by a chemical that comes out of the body and smells like dead fish. Could there be a *reason* for her problem? Another excited click brought her to the TMAU Foundation, where a sympathetic new friend referred Camille to Dr. George Preti, one of the few experts in the world on the disorder, at Philadelphia's Monell Chemical Senses Institute.

Preti was able to diagnose Camille—a classic case. She was relieved after all the years of wondering what was wrong with her that she had a name and cause for her condition. But she was also angry.

"I was pissed," she says. "I was mad at the world. I mean really, really, really angry. 'Why has this happened to me? I have two siblings; neither one of them has it. Why me?'"

HOLD THE CHOLINE, PLEASE!

Unfortunately, there is no medical answer to Camille's question: why me? The enzyme deficiency that plagues her is genetic: the luck of the draw, something she was born with. But it could certainly explain why TMAU makes you smell bad.

Preti describes TMAU as a metabolic disorder. The enzyme that metabolizes a chemical called trimethylamine (TMA) is not working correctly. You may never have heard of it, but TMA is inside your body right now, produced in everyone's large intestines by the bacteria that live there. The bacteria get it from our food, particularly foods that contain choline. Choline's a pretty ordinary chemical unless you have TMAU—in which case it becomes your own personal Darth Vader. The choline makes TMA, and your enzyme deficiency means that the TMA doesn't get broken down.

"In individuals with this disorder, this enzyme is not working at peak capacity because of genetics," says Preti. "Because trimethylamine *is* a volatile chemical, it will come out through the sweat, spit, and other body secretions." Even your breath carries it. And trimethylamine smells terrible.

Preti says in documented cases more women than men are affected, and he's not sure why that is. Again, it might be because women are more likely to seek treatment for medical conditions than men are. Or perhaps there's less of a social stigma attached to men that smell bad.

In most people, enzymes convert 95 to 100 percent of their naturally occurring TMA to the more soluble and less smelly trimethylamine-oxide—and it's excreted in your urine. It's undetectable. But people with TMAU have all that TMA circulating through the body; even so, only about 10 percent of the one hundred or so people Preti has diagnosed with TMAU have the fishy odor. And let's make it a little *more* complicated: the people who *do* smell don't smell all the time. The symptoms tend to flare after what Preti calls "a choline challenge."

Just about every food available—eggs, meats, many types of beans, milk, cheese, bread, and, of course, fish—contains choline. When someone with TMAU eats a high-choline food, trimethylamine builds up in the body.

Preti has helped Camille design a highly restricted diet of mostly fresh fruits and vegetables to ward off the accumulation of TMA in her system.

"It's working," Camille says. "Thank God for that. For breakfast I have a banana, sometimes a kiwi. I eat these rye crisps in very limited amount with apple butter on them. For lunch, celery, carrots, cucumber, sometimes a mango. I started having turkey breast from a special deli so that I know that the bird was raised very purely. Dinner is a hard one. It's just a repeat of lunch."

A strict diet is only one of the routines Camille has developed to try to keep the odor at bay. She takes chlorophyll tablets every day, which help her digestion. And, as a purely practical solution, she showers over and over again.

"I wash with several different products and I scrub very hard," says Camille. "I use two different kinds of deodorant. And a lot of perfume. Before I actually leave the house, I spray all of my clothes with Febreze, all up and down. And I also spray my feet and my socks." She feels she can cope now—because of the Internet friendship that led her to Dr. Preti.

THE TMAU FOUNDATION

Sandy Gordon is the woman who helped Camille on the Internet. She also suffers from trimethylaminuria, and did something about it, founding and running the TMAU Foundation.

Sandy's was a late-onset case: she was in her early thirties when her body became unable to metabolize TMA. Of course, it took several years before she became aware of it—who would suspect that they gave off a sudden, dreadful odor? In fact, she remembers even calling the maintenance man to her New York City apartment to check her bathroom.

"It just smelled horribly," she recalls. "I thought maybe there was some kind of a problem with the sewer."

It wasn't the sewer. It was Sandy. Her search for that elusive TMAU diagnosis not only took years, it took her life savings.

"I literally spent $27,000 of my own money," she says. "I had eight different unnecessary surgeries."

It was a dentist who saved her. Sandy's breath made him suspect TMAU. He sent her to Philadelphia's Monell Institute and Preti.

Sandy endured the same kinds of painful social ostracism as Camille. She says that many people with the condition are afraid to form relationships—to put themselves "out there."

"For a long time I backed away from wanting to socialize," says Sandy. "I have such a large, rambunctious family. They just wanted me to participate. They thought it was really silly that I wanted to exclude myself. I remember my sister was having an event. I said: 'I'm coming to help you, but then I'm leaving. I'm not staying.' And she said: 'Stop making excuses. It's always about *you*. It shouldn't be, because it's *my* party. You're my sister, and if you smell, that's fine. Those who are offended—let them leave. But I want you to be there.'"

Camille felt that Sandy had, in a very real way, saved her life, but they'd never met. We brought Sandy and Camille together. Just before they were introduced, we realized that Camille had never even met anyone else with TMAU.

We invited them both to our offices—and it's no exaggeration to say that they clung to each other. There were some tears—then some astonishment as Sandy dumped out a bag she had brought with her—bottle after bottle of prescription medication given to her, all for conditions she didn't have, because a diagnosis of TMAU is so rare that most doctors miss it.

Camille credits Sandy and the foundation for turning her life around, giving her a desperately needed source of support. She knows now that she is no longer alone. Still, what both she and Sandy most want, a cure, remains elusive.

ENZYME REPLACEMENT

You might wonder, like we did, why there isn't some kind of pill or shot to give TMAU sufferers the enzyme they need. That's normally the way that liver enzyme issues are resolved—with enzyme replacement therapy.

Because of the rarity of the disorder, however, there simply hasn't been the money to pursue a cure.

"Unfortunately, because there's less than a thousand people in the world that have been officially diagnosed with trimethylaminuria, the money isn't there," says Sandy. "There's not really much of an incentive for coming up with the enzyme replacement. The pharmaceutical companies are not going to dump a bunch of time and effort into that because less than a thousand people will buy the enzyme in the end."

The foundation is trying to enlist the help of doctors, researchers, and chemical companies to find a cure. They're advocating for more testing for the disorder, which they think is underreported. In other words, they think there are a lot more Camilles out there, suffering without knowing what's wrong, or afraid to get tested because of the stigma attached to having a condition that causes such an unpleasant odor.

"There is no cure right now, because it is a genetic disorder," says Preti. "The only way to fully cure an individual who has it is to do genetic engineering, and that is not on the immediate horizon as far as I can see."

Both Sandy and Camille try to remain upbeat.

"We can't let it be our whole existence," says Sandy. "We're going to lick this thing."

. . .

CAMILLE HAS PROMISED HERSELF she will use her experience to make something positive happen. Remember, she's a teacher, and though she knows that not many children will suffer from TMAU, she is working on a school curriculum to help children who are different in *any* way, so they won't have to endure the ridicule she once did. And now that she finally has a diagnosis, she has told her boyfriend what the problem is. She no longer hides herself away, and her special diet makes her condition more bearable.

"We're trying to work things out," she says. "And I feel very positive about that. There's hope."

Perhaps you'll come away from our brush with TMAU with the same thought that we did: amazement at the sheer power of *having a diagnosis*. Just knowing what is wrong seems to be a powerful key to recuperation. Allow us fifteen seconds on the soapbox: if you have your own medical mystery, go see a doctor. When it comes to your own body, knowledge is power.

4. FACE BLINDNESS

THEY ARE COMPLETELY SANE, COMPLETELY FUNCTIONAL. THEY can look at a photograph of a nose and know what it is. They recognize an eye when they see it. Chins, eyebrows—individually, as objects, they make sense. But as soon as you combine them into a face? For these people, it all goes blank.

It seems like the premise of a science fiction plot, or a great beginning to a surreal short story: people who can't "see" human faces. Even if you accept that it's real (which took me a while to do), you jump to a completely incorrect conclusion: it has to be some sort of psychological syndrome, right? People who don't "want" to see other people? Some people have an incredibly bad memory for names. Why not faces?

Nope.

The problem is neurological—a connection somewhere in the brain that just isn't happening. It's called prosopagnosia, and people who have it are called "face blind." When you combine eyes, nose, mouth, chin—you see a face. For prosopagnosiacs, it's a mysterious blank.

A SEA OF FACES

People with "proso," as they call it, aren't even that hard to find. Heather Sellers, for instance, is an English professor at Hope College in Holland, Michigan. She's also an author who has written about her condition—her new book is called *Face First*. She's heard that some people "never forget a face," but she is blind to them, even the faces of those nearest and dearest to her.

The instant someone leaves her sight, the image of his or her face quickly fades. Heather has an excellent memory for names, phone numbers, and the obscure details of the texts she teaches. But, mysteriously, she is unable to retain faces. Even her own image in a mirror throws her off.

"I've been in a situation where there is just a sea of faces that are reflected [in a mirror]," she says. "I won't know which one is me! It's frightening and confusing, really disorienting. I thought I was crazy. My students, when they go to Japan, come back and say, 'Everybody looked the same!' That's how I feel here. I have people that I see regularly. Colleagues. And they are all standing there in front of me. It would be like you standing in front of twenty dogs from your neighborhood, all of them golden retrievers."

Heather relies on clues like clothing, hair, height, gait, or the sound of a voice to help her figure out who people are.

"I wouldn't be able to recognize my mother if she was walking down the street," says Heather. "And then, along with that, I mistake people for her."

. . .

GROWING UP, Heather says she not only had trouble making friends in school but even recognizing the ones she had.

"I would put them in groups: the redheaded kids, and the brown-headed kids, and the curly-haired kids. I always knew there was something wrong, but I had no idea what it was."

The problem plagued her through high school and into her adult life. Not recognizing coworkers has often strained her professional relationships and damaged her career.

"I avoided committee meetings and a lot of my duties at my college, because it was so confusing to go into a room after five years and still not know who these people were."

After she was married, Heather says she often lost her husband when they'd shop for groceries. During the 5K road races they ran, she would memorize the registration number pinned to his shirt so she could find him in a crowd.

Her prosopagnosia has caused her to move approximately every five years. She felt that the embarrassment of not recognizing people was just too great. She would feel enormous relief and gratitude when she'd move into a new community—it meant people would introduce themselves to her. Everyone was a stranger, and she wasn't expected to remember who anybody was.

DIAGNOSING THE DISORDER

Nancy Kanwisher, who investigates visual perception and cognition in a brain research laboratory that she runs at MIT, notes that until recently most prosopagnosia cases she

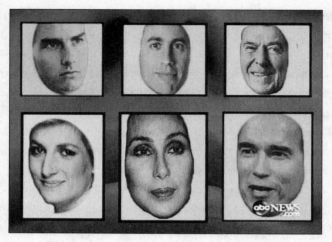

How many of these celebrities can you identify?
Turn the page for answers.

studied were the result of a stroke or a brain injury. But recent research indicates that far more people are *born* with
prosopagnosia than develop it from injury or illness. In fact,
experts now estimate approximately 2 percent of the population may have some degree of face blindness—it's about as
common as dyslexia. There may be a single, dominant gene
to blame (which means a child may inherit the disorder even
if only one parent has it).

Psychology professor Ken Nakayama, who heads the Prosopagnosia Research Center at Harvard University, has created a number of face perception tests to diagnose people
who think they may have the disorder. Nakayama typically
tests whole families for memory and perception if one member of that family presents with symptoms of face blindness.
One test he uses involves images of celebrity heads—bald. It's
a telltale trait for people with prosopagnosia; they can recall

hair, even though facial features instantly evaporate from their memories.

One family Nakayama tested, the Heards, recognized, on average, only nineteen out of the sixty famous faces. Most of us (without "proso") can identify about fifty-three.

Nakayama has a personal interest in all this—he and his wife think that he is mildly prosopagnosic himself. Their clue? He can't "follow" some movies, another trait among people who have proso. As the characters on screen change outfits and hairstyles, he becomes confused by the faces disappearing and reappearing, can't keep them straight, and loses the thread of the story.

THE HEARD FAMILY

Catherine Heard, who lives outside Toronto, is one daughter in that family that remembered only nineteen of the sixty faces. She, too, often finds films baffling, especially American ones.

"The actors are all really good-looking," she says, "and they look generic. Recently, I was in a supermarket. On the magazines by the checkout there were photos of two blond actresses. I thought: 'These women look exactly the same to me. I can't tell them apart.' I do much better with foreign films where the actors look less beautiful. Especially British films. The teeth are, you know . . ."

Catherine, an artist, can't paint faces from memory, can't "see" them in her head. But there's nothing wrong with her other memories: she can, for example, recall every visual detail of Monet's *Water Lilies* paintings.

Jim Heard, Catherine's father, a retired art teacher who is also prosopagnosic, says the disorder has become more poignant with age: "I would like to be able to remember my wife's face, for example, or my father's face, who's dead, but I don't. It's sad to lose that recollection." The framed photos of relatives that cover your bureau? Virtually meaningless to a prosopagnosiac.

Like just about everyone else with proso, Jim has spent his life *pretending* to recognize faces. "You hide it," he says. "I recognize people; it's just faces I don't recognize. I recognize voices, the way somebody walks. All those kinds of little things that you put together that make a person an individual."

Jim's other daughter, Jayne Kalmar, lives in Winnipeg. A neuroscientist with two young children, she is also face-blind. She remembers one way her dad coped with the disorder. Her mother would often cue Jim: "Mom would tell Dad, 'Oh, that's one of your students.'"

Jim never had a clue that he had a neurological disorder. He just knew that he, along with his daughters, seemed to have a terrible time recognizing faces. He blamed himself and felt inadequate and guilty. "I thought it was me, and that I wasn't paying attention," he says. "I didn't have a clue as to why I was like that."

It was Jayne who told the family what was going on, after an upsetting incident that would make any parent wince: when she went to her son Gabriel's day-care center, she picked up the wrong child.

ANSWERS TO CELEBRITY PROSOPAGNOSIA TEST:
Top row: Tom Cruise, Jerry Seinfeld, Ronald Reagan
Bottom row: Princess Diana, Cher, Arnold Schwarzenegger

"My son was about maybe ten months old," says Jayne. "The children were all out in the playground. It was a little windy so they had hoods up. All I had to work with was the face—no hair clues. Babies don't have a lot of strong facial features that stand out. If you can just memorize one part of a face, you're okay. There was a little baby that I was walking towards. I thought it was Gabriel, and the baby cooed and smiled at me. He responded to me, which reinforced my belief that it was my son. I went over to him. The day-care women were watching. I turned to them and said, 'Why doesn't he have his own jacket on? I brought Gabriel in a jacket this morning.' They were waiting to see if there was a joke. Some people looked a little horrified. I continued to talk to him and play with him—and then I got a sense that something wasn't right. I picked him up and took off his hood. I was staring really hard, in a panic, and feeling embarrassed, and eventually had to ask if he was my child. The parent/child relationship is supposed to be the strongest bond. I was fortunate because my daughter had been at that day care for four years, and these women knew me well."

After failing to recognize her own son, Jayne began a desperate search to find out what was wrong with her. She went online and began researching terms like "facial recognition" and "disorder," which eventually brought her and her family to Nakayama.

CHILDREN AND PROSOPAGNOSIA

Depression and shame are unfortunately often two of the most common symptoms of prosopagnosia. Nakayama has observed that it is often children with the disorder who have the hardest time coping. "They think they're stupid," he says. "They're ashamed. You go to the playground and you can't recognize other kids or your sisters or your brothers. And it's very disturbing, but you can't talk to other people because they won't understand you. How's a parent to know their kid can't recognize faces?"

Nakayama adds that the vast majority of pediatricians have never heard of the disorder, let alone parents. "People who study child development have probably never even heard of the word," he says. "You get tested for ADHD, you get tested for dyslexia. There's no test in school for this." Nakayama notes that many kids on the autism spectrum are probably prosopagnosic.

In high school, Heather gravitated toward people who had obvious physical differences, because she could recognize them. "I liked the girl in the wheelchair. The really overweight guy. My high school boyfriend had the disorder that causes men to bald at age fifteen—and he had a beard down to here!" She laughs. "And I think now it's because I could find him. That's the only guy I could *find* in the whole school!"

THE NEUROLOGY OF PROSOPAGNOSIA

Nakayama says the disorder was first identified in 1947 by a German neurologist who identified three people with brain lesions who had prosopagnosia. It wasn't until the mid-1990s that researchers identified the developmental, congenital type of prosopagnosia—the kind that afflicts Heather Sellers and the Heards.

In Nancy Kanwisher's lab at MIT, researchers began MRI brain scans on people who were congenital prosopagnosiacs. The researchers were particularly interested in the region of the brain that has to do with facial recognition. "This particular region in the right hemisphere, near the bottom of the brain, is where you'll find a little patch—about a half a cubic centimeter," says Kanwisher. "We call that region the fusiform face area. We've been studying it for about ten years. We know that it responds very strongly when you look at faces, much more strongly than when you look at any other kind of object."

Kanwisher and fellow researchers believe this might be the area of our brain that evolved to differentiate faces from all other visual clues; a vital evolutionary skill. It hardwires us to find faces—it's the reason that you "see" a face when you look at the headlights and grille of a car, or at an electric socket, with its "eyes" and "mouth."

Kanwisher says that she and her team have noticed that the face-selective regions are smaller in the developmental prosopagnosic subjects than in normal subjects, but that they haven't done enough testing to know if that's a significant discovery. The fusiform region responds fairly normally in prosopagnosiacs, and Kanwisher has no idea why its size should affect facial recognition.

"It leaves us with a real scientific puzzle," she says. "Either that region is not functioning normally, or it is working normally and the signal is just not getting out of that region of the brain to other areas where it needs to go. Or we're all way off base and that isn't the crux of face recognition, in that part of the brain, in the first place, and the real action is somewhere else."

The latest studies, using MRIs to look at the communication pathways in the brain, show that people with proso have some disruptions in how the brain talks to itself; an inability to put the pieces together when it comes to faces.

Although Nakayama cautions that segmenting the brain into parts that have exclusive "functions" may be misleading, he says prosopagnosia supports that view. "Some people refer to [the brain] as one giant piece of green cheese, all functions mixed together," he says. "Or separate little modules of different functions. Prosopagnosia makes you think there's special little functions."

Nakayama thinks the condition is probably genetic, but the dominant gene that causes it has yet to be identified. He studied one large family of prosopagnosiacs: eight brothers and sisters, a mother and a father, and a maternal uncle.

"It probably is some kind of neurological disorder," he says. "I don't even want to call it a disorder. It's a variation in human ability. And it exists on a really wide spectrum. There are people who just occasionally have trouble. And then there are other people who have trouble all the time."

Mild prosopagnosiacs can train themselves to memorize a limited number of faces, but there is no known treatment for the condition at this time. Computers may be able to help people recognize faces at some point, but Nakayama thinks that is still a distant hope: "Computers aren't very good at recognizing somebody's face in different lighting conditions and expressions," says Nakayama. "But they may in ten, twenty years. Who knows?"

COMING OUT OF THE CLOSET

The Heard family and Heather Sellers were vastly relieved to give a label to a condition that had plagued them all their lives. "I'm so happy to have a name, something to call it," says Heather. "But if you could send me over to MIT today and fix my brain, I'd have to think really a long time. I like some of the things that it gives me. I like that I focus on who the person is. I'm not distracted by appearances."

Heather has learned to cope by using other clues: recognizing people by their clothing, jewelry, or gait, how they sit, stand, act—even by their smell! "I have one very dear friend who wears patchouli," she says. "I don't really care for the scent. But I love that she wears it, because I always know it's Jackie. Jackie is coming! I smell her before I see her."

Nakayama speculates that in recent centuries, prosopagnosia probably wasn't that much of a deficit. "People lived in a small town," he says, "and they knew all their neighbors. In the old days, we had two outfits, and so you could recognize people. Each social class had to have a different kind of outfit. Today we have a very complicated society. People have got lots of clothing. Our society is fast and chaotic."

Nakayama says that one of the greater mysteries of the condition is this: many prosopagnosiacs who can't "see" the face can still process subtle information about it. They can tell whether it is happy, sad, angry, puzzled. They can often detect ethnicity, gender—even beauty.

But Heather worries about the friendships she has lost by passing people on the street and not recognizing them.

"It's been reported back to me—'She's so aloof,'" says Heather. "'She's so stuck up.'"

Heather's diagnosis changed her life. She's no longer ashamed of her prosopagnosia. "Now that I'm out," says Heather, "if I'm meeting somebody new, I say, 'I'm not able to recognize people. I won't recognize you. You'll always have to identify yourself.'"

Jim has learned the hard way that a face is something that is "very, very personal. It's *you*. And if you don't remember somebody who thinks you should know them, that's kind of an insult—either you're not important enough for me to remember or you're eminently forgettable."

As in Heather's case, Jim's diagnosis has made an enormous difference in his life. It has set him free.

"If you're faking a relationship with people all the time," Jim says, "and then all of a sudden have to acknowledge this to yourself or others, that's kind of coming out. You have to admit to other people you don't know them. It's quite liberating."

I'll bet after reading this chapter, you have an urge to go to the mirror and take a long, hard look at yourself. And I would hope it will make you feel less embarrassed when you can't remember someone you've met before—after all, it may just be your brain playing tricks on you.

5. THE COLOR OF SOUND

THE NOTORIOUS NINETEENTH-CENTURY FRENCH POET ARTHUR Rimbaud wrote: "A black, E white, I red, U green, O blue." It's one of the most famous historical examples of a bizarre medical mystery: synesthesia, a crossing of the senses or, literally, "joined sensation." For this poet, letters were synonymous with colors—A *was* black, E *was* white. And for Rimbaud, synesthesia was a gift. It unlocked metaphor, gave him another way of "seeing" words, and was a poetic technique used by the French symbolist movement as part of their practice of the "derangement of the senses."

Today, however, on the other side of the Channel, London pub owner James Wannerton, now in his late forties, considers his synesthesia to be a nuisance. It's been with him all his life. James *tastes* almost every word he hears, even the words of his customers' orders.

"The problem I have," he says, "is somebody will come in and order, say, a 'pint' of that. I get the bacon rind taste. They'll order a packet of 'roasted nuts.' I don't get 'roasted nuts'; I get some sort of peculiar meat taste."

For him, "Covent Garden" tastes of chocolate; the words "dad" and "mum" come with flavors. As if that's not odd enough, the name "Derrick" is highly unpleasant for James. "It's horrible. Earwax!" he says.

Synesthesia was one of the few medical mysteries that leapt to mind when we first embarked on the series. I'd always been fascinated by it—I think because I was mildly synesthetic as a child. Names seemed to have "colors" to me—and the colors were remarkably consistent. I named my dolls as much by what color the name was as anything else. I had pretty much forgotten about it (names had become just names by the time I was in junior high) until I read an article about synesthesia when I was in college—and had a feeling of recognition.

A COMMON PHENOMENON

So, what *color* is the number eight? What does Swiss cheese *sound* like? It turns out seeing (or tasting) sounds, numbers, or letters is not as uncommon as you might think. Medical experts estimate that one in twenty-three people have synesthesia. And there are different varieties—crossovers between sight, taste, touch, and hearing.

"What's happening in a synesthete's brain is that neighboring neural areas have more cross talk than normal," says Dr. David Eagleman of the University of Texas Medical School in Houston. "There are two parts of the brain, and they're talking to each other. That causes the activity of one area to trigger the activity of the other area. Letters might trigger a color."

Eagleman says that synesthesia appears to be inherited: "We're finding big families where synesthesia runs through the tree, and then we're zooming in on the genes responsible for that. We have the technology to really follow this up and try to find the gene or genes involved in synesthesia. That's what my laboratory is doing."

While some people might think that people who say they "see" or "taste" sounds are speaking metaphorically, or even making it all up, Eagleman says modern research techniques have dispelled that notion: "We know from several different angles, including the neuroimaging, genetics, and behavioral tests . . . that synesthesia is a real thing." And it's consistent—if a sound is a particular shade of green, it will always stay that way.

Take Laura Rosser's case. Yes, she sees specific colors when she looks at black letters or numbers on a white page—always the same colors. But Laura also sees colors when she plays notes on a piano. The note B is sparkling silver. And D flat? "Wondrous, pure periwinkle," she says. "E flat is turquoise. Very warm turquoise."

Dr. Randolph Blake of Vanderbilt University explains: "That's a real color experience that's as vivid and as real as the colors that you and I see ordinarily in the world. It's just that it's being evoked in a highly unusual way."

Blake agreed to let us peek inside Laura Rosser's brain to see synesthesia in action—a brain scan of her occipital lobe. As black letters flashed before her eyes inside the scanning machine, Laura recorded the colors she saw. And amazingly, real-time images of her brain's reactions when she's looking at the letters show that the *color* areas are active, areas that would not light up in a normal brain. "We think that there are some unusually strong connections between areas of her brain that aren't so strongly connected in our brains," says

Blake. "So strong that when she's looking at a letter, it actually automatically activates that color area."

Eagleman says that brain-imaging research into synesthesia has caused a paradigm shift in science and forced a fundamental rethinking about how the brain is organized. "Sensory channels are not as separate as we once thought that they were," he says. "And the idea that the brain is modular is not true in any more than a general way. The other sense of a paradigm shift is personal: synesthesia highlights the amazing differences in the way people see the same thing, reminding us that each brain filters out the world in its own uniquely subjective way. So the world is far more subjective than objective—and synesthesia heightens our sensitivity to diversity and difference."

WE'RE ALL SYNESTHETIC

Most people would agree that louder tones are "brighter" than softer tones, and lower tones are both "larger" and "darker" than high ones. That's a form of synesthesia. In our sense of smell, the same rules seem to apply. We say, for example, that a darkly tinted liquid tastes and smells stronger than a liquid that is pale. When we dance, we are doing what researchers call "cross-sensory mapping" in which our body rhythms translate sound rhythms, both visually and kinetically.

Dr. Richard Cytowic of George Washington University is a leading neurologist in this field. He gives a classic example of the ways in which everyone's brain works synesthetically. Look at the illustrations on the next page.

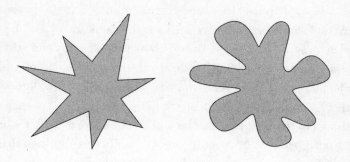

Booba and Kikki. Which one's which?

"In alien Martian language," says Cytowic, "one shape is a booba and the other one is a kikki. Which one is the spike shape and which is the blob's shape? Ninety-eight percent of people, no matter what language they speak, pick the jagged shape as kikki because the visual jags imitate the 'kikki' sound and the sharp motor inflection of the tongue against the palate. Whereas the blob's visual contours are more like the sound and motor inflections of 'booba.' And what this shows is that in biology, preexisting patterns are often co-opted, so that synesthetic associations our ancestors made long ago have grown into the more abstract kinds of language that we have today. And this is why metaphors make sense."

Synesthesia has long been associated with metaphor in poetry and may, in fact, be at least part of what is at the root of the kind of metaphoric language in verse. John Keats in his famous poem "Ode to a Nightingale" asks for a wine "Tasting of Flora and the country green,/Dance, and Provençal song, and sunburnt mirth . . ." In other words, wine that tastes of color, motion, sound, and heat.

"What happens in a synesthete's brain is actually just an example of what happens in normal brains also," Dr. Eagleman says. "So, for example with metaphor, every time that you connect two dissimilar domains and make some sort of metaphor that connects them, that's essentially what a synesthete's brain is doing all of the time. And there are many things in the language that we understand, like a 'loud' tie or 'sharp' cheese or a 'sweet' personality. These are things that are essentially synesthetically generated metaphors but our brains understand them somehow. Again, indicating that that sort of cross-wiring is present in normal brains."

Cytowic says that Braille is a clear example of how synesthesia is a universal human inclination. "When newly blind people learn to read Braille, the brain area corresponding to the reading finger greatly expands," he says. "Tactile connections into the unused visual cortex strengthen, changing its functional assignment from seeing to feeling Braille and reading it. Even more remarkably, when sighted people are blindfolded for just two days, their visual cortex undergoes a functional reassignment, suddenly responding to sounds, to touch, and to words. So the sudden ability of the brain to 'see with the ears and the fingers' shows that these connections exist within all of us."

"We're all synesthetic," Cytowic adds. "The difference between normal and synesthetic brains is not whether there's cross talk, but how much cross talk there is. 'Colored hearing' is very common, where sound, ordinary environmental sounds—dog barks, slamming doors, cars—will cause an experience of something like fireworks, and colored shapes arise. They move around a little bit, and one fades away to be replaced by another one, as long as the sound continues, like in a kaleidoscopic montage."

And it's not a passing event: "A defining feature [of the condition] is that once synesthetic associations are established in childhood, the links stay fixed for life," says Cytowic.

SPATIAL SEQUENCE SYNESTHESIA

It's not just colors and letters—in what's called spatial sequence synesthesia, a synesthete will perceive the days of the week or the months of the year as having particular spatial locations. It's actually one of the most common forms of the condition. Ask sisters Trish Goodwin and Molly Altobelli—they live in Texas and are helping with Dr. Eagleman's research in Houston. The sisters first figured out around the dinner table that they and their mother perceived numbers in a different way. Dad, of course, thought of numbers as small black marks on a page. Not the women—for them, numbers floated in space and had different sizes and different positions.

"My sisters and I and my parents were talking at dinner one night," says Trish, "and were comparing how numbers were in certain different places, or we thought of them in a sort of bending line. And we would all just sort of say, 'Oh, yeah, I know what you mean but mine is different because it goes like this and it goes like this.' And my dad looked at us and went, 'You guys are crazy, what are you even talking about? Numbers aren't on a line. They're just numbers.' That's when we realized it was a little bit odd."

"I thought my dad was crazy," says Molly. "It was four against one. All four of us knew what we were talking about. *He* seemed like the odd one out."

Eagleman has used 3-D computer software to construct the spatial "number world" the sisters describe. "Trish had her weekdays arranged on the floor around her feet," says Eagleman. "Molly has her weekdays floating up in space. And the same with numbers. Trish has her numbers along the ground, whereas Molly's numbers are floating up along the left side of her body, way up into the middle of the air."

Eagleman has been searching for the genetic link for synesthesia in part by looking at Molly and Trish's family. Molly invited Eagleman to get samples for his genetic study at her wedding.

"We had all this family in town for the wedding," says Molly. "They were all together at our aunt and uncle's house. The researchers handed out a bunch of questionnaires about synesthesia to figure out who had it. They took saliva samples so that they could do DNA tests," to try to find where on the DNA strand synesthesia might show up.

Eagleman says his "wedding crashing" paid off. He and his team made a discovery. "By collecting their DNA and then looking at how the synesthesia goes through the family and what changes in their DNA follow that, we were able to find a region" in the gene that carries the trait, he says.

Cytowic adds that he thinks synesthesia is the result of a genetic mutation. "A fetus makes two million synapses a second, giving newborns an excess of working connections among brain areas," he says. "These are then pruned away to leave the modular organization that we know of in adults. So the hypothesis says that inheriting a genetic mutation leads to a failure to prune excess connections that ordinarily would've been eliminated by synaptic competition early in life. What the mutation confers then is *hyper*connectivity—wherever it's expressed in the brain. When [certain types of] synesthetes look at a letter, they also activate the color area of the brain called 'V-4.' And they do this because the areas are hyper-connected thanks to inheriting a genetic mutation."

Normally, synesthesia works as a one-way street. So, for example, sound goes to color in "colored hearing," but color doesn't go to sound. The handful of people who have it in both directions sometimes are overwhelmed by it. Eighty percent of synesthetes experience the phenomenon in a second or third area, which leads researchers to think that they have the gene that causes synesthesia expressed in two or three different areas of their brains.

It's fascinating stuff, but why would scientists spend so much time putting synesthetes under the microscope?

"One of the reasons we're studying synesthesia is because we're trying to determine how the normal brain integrates signals from all of the different senses," says Eagleman. "The brain has to find a balance between integrating those signals so that it sees a unified picture of the world, and also keeping them separate so that it knows what belongs to what. So we're trying to figure out how the normal brain does this, and that's why it's very useful for us to look at the synesthetic brain."

Cytowic adds: "I see it leading us to new ways of seeing how the brain is organized. That the senses cooperate and are connected with each other far more than we thought that they were. It used to be that by definition the brain was seen as modular. Each module was insulated. There was no leakiness to other modules. Now we know that the brain is very leaky. All of us are making cross-sensory mappings all the time. For example, when you listen to me speak, you're also lip-reading. What you see helps you hear."

THE GIFT OF SYNESTHESIA

"Across the board, synesthetes are very happy that they have synesthesia," Eagleman notes. "They consider it something of a gift. And as far as we can tell from a neuroscience point of view, there's no disadvantage to it. In fact, it seems advantageous, because it helps people to tag things in different dimensions. So, for example, if you have colored numbers and you're remembering somebody's phone number, you not only have the sequence of numbers, but now you have colors that might help as a memory aid."

Cywotic concurs. He says synesthetes "love" their gift of being able to hear colors or taste sounds. "Very, very few people are disturbed by it," he says. "It helps you remember things. Synesthetes do, in fact, have extraordinarily good memories. One of the gifts of synesthesia is heightened creativity, especially the capacity for metaphor. But what if this gene for hyperconnectivity, for cross talk, were expressed not selectively here and there, but diffusely in somebody's brain? Then you'd have a heightened ability to link seemingly different things. And that's a definition of metaphor, isn't it? Seeing the similar in the dissimilar and linking seemingly different things in creative ways. We've long known that synesthesia is much more common in creative people like artists and composers. Some famous synesthetes include the novelist

Vladimir Nabokov, the composer Stevie Wonder, and paint-ers David Hockney and Wassily Kandinsky."

Cytowic has found that synesthetes, as a rule, are more open to experience than other people. "They're less con-strained," he says. "They just have a more general open atti-tude towards life because they're used to mapping one concept to another in unconventional ways."

Laura Rosser is convinced that synesthesia enhances ex-perience rather than detracts from it. As she plays the piano, she sees a flood of color. "I see [synesthesia] as a gift, as a sort of spiritual 'God thing' that enables more intuition, to be able to see some extra things out there."

A life without it?

"It would be like going from seeing everything in color to a world that was monochromatic," Laura says.

AFTER WE FINISHED producing the show, I was sad that my childhood synesthesia had somehow, when I wasn't look-ing, drifted away. I now live in that world Laura wouldn't want to inhabit—a world in which this page is just . . . black and white.

6. SEXSOMNIA

IF YOUR FIRST REACTION TO THIS SYNDROME IS "YEAH, SURE," you're not alone. When one of our producers brought it up, there were some raised eyebrows at the table. Turns out, sadly, that this is an attitude that most of the patients encounter as well. After all, "Yes, I grabbed you and had sex with you, but I was asleep at the time" strikes anyone as unusual, to say the least. But doctors, believe it or not, have a name for the act of sex while asleep—sexsomnia.

In the five years since they've been married, Tyson Otts, a factory worker in South Carolina, has routinely initiated sex with his wife when he is fast asleep. Like many of the patients we interviewed who were faced with unusual diagnoses, Tyson and his wife were willing to talk to us about this most private event to make sure that other people who suffer wouldn't be alone.

NOT POSSIBLE?

Tyson's own wife had trouble believing that her husband was truly asleep when he would come on to her in the middle of night.

"I could see where she would think I wasn't sleeping," says Tyson. "But I promise you, I am."

Tyson says that he has absolutely no idea *why* he'd have sex with his wife while he's sleeping. "It is nothing that I'm dreaming about that I can remember," he says. "It's just natural reaction or instinct or something like that."

His wife, Vanessa, says Tyson will roll over in bed and start kissing her and trying to rip off her clothes. Vanessa has mixed feelings about her husband's vigorous foreplay. "I wish he would know he was doing it, because [it's] a really big turn-on," she laughs. "I mean, not if he's gonna choke me or whatever; but, you know, being more aggressive."

Here's the problem: Vanessa ends up hot, bothered, and unsatisfied. "We never get to the point of sex," she laments. "Then he falls back to sleep. It's disappointing. I can't wake him up, and I can't turn him on. I've tried that."

Tyson, on the other hand, fails to see what's erotic about his behavior. He says one night Vanessa told him that he held her down as he began to force himself on her. "That really scared me," says Tyson. "I just don't think that's appropriate behavior. It's way out of character [for me] to be holding somebody down against their will."

Vanessa is a bit more sanguine. "It didn't scare me at all when he did it," she says. "I was, like, oh wow! He's being kind of freaky tonight."

Dr. Mike Mangen, a research psychologist at the University of New Hampshire, says that people are often incredulous when they hear about sexsomnia. "The knee-jerk response is to say, no way, it's not possible," he says. "But people walk in their sleep. They talk in their sleep. People do all kinds of crazy things in their sleep. And it just hasn't entered the popular mind that sexual behavior can be just another type of sleep behavior."

Mangen and others have been focusing their research efforts on the underlying causes of the disorder, which seems to originate in a disconnect between two parts of our brains—one area with the primal urge for sex, and the other, the brain's cortex, which controls rationality and judgment. "Basically what you have is a sexually motivated brain and body and a cortex that is switched off," says Mangen. "When [the cortex] is switched off, you have a sexually activated body that's having its way."

Researchers think that sexsomnia is one of a spectrum of sleep disorders (called parasomnias) that include sleepwalking and talking in your sleep. But parasomnias can also include behaviors that are sexual and violent. Sexsomnia is clearly unusual, but researchers say the reported number of cases may be low because most people don't think it's a condition they can do anything about, and maybe they don't even know it's a medical problem. Barring running a sleep study in a lab (called polysomnography), it's pretty difficult to document. Sleep lab cameras have given video evidence that patients, asleep by all measures of their brain waves, perform all sorts of parasomnias, but without a diagnosis from a sleep specialist, people with sexsomnia generally suffer through it without even knowing there's a diagnosis.

BUT WHAT IF IT GETS VIOLENT?

For Lori and Bob Norman, also of South Carolina, it's not sex. They have become accidental combatants in a nocturnal prizefight. Repeatedly during their nine-year marriage, a sleep disorder has caused Bob to unwittingly assault his wife.

"I woke up with him pounding the pillow right beside my face," says Lori. "I mean, within inches of my face. We're sound asleep and he takes his two hands with his fists together and pounds me on the back of the neck. And I just screamed and threw my hands up over my head and grabbed his hands as they were coming down again."

Bob insists his nocturnal behavior is completely out of character. "I've been meditating for thirty-five years," he says. "I think of myself as healthy and peaceful."

But on the nights when there is violence in the Normans' bedroom, Bob often finds that he wakes up from strange dreams that are sometimes reminiscent of the films of Alfred Hitchcock.

"I'm watching a flock of ducks in the water," says Bob of one such dream. "And at some point they started coming towards me. I just had this knowing that I was in danger—that they were going to attack me."

The impending attack in Bob's dream played out in the Normans' bed. "I was sound asleep and he suddenly kicked me really hard," says Lori.

REM BEHAVIOR DISORDER

Bob has been diagnosed with REM (rapid eye movement) behavior disorder or RBD, a condition that occurs in the dreaming stage of sleep. It's another variation of parasomnia—one in which the sleeper can be awakened and will immediately recall vivid, often violent dreams.

Dr. Nancy Foldvary, who directs the Sleep Disorders Center at the Cleveland Clinic, says: "In REM sleep, interestingly, the brain is very active. We dream." And while we dream, our brain takes care to paralyze most of our muscles. "That's the normal state of REM. It's almost a protective effect to be paralyzed so that we cannot move during that state."

But for people with REM behavior disorder, the natural mechanism that causes paralysis during sleep fails. "They thrash around," says Foldvary. "They may consider the wife an enemy. They're acting out a dream."

Significantly, researchers have linked the odd behaviors of RBD to other even more serious neurodegenerative disorders like Parkinson's disease. "What is clearly coming out is that REM disorder appears eight to ten to fifteen years before patients develop Parkinson's disease," says Foldvary.

Bob finds this research unsettling, to say the least. "It could be extremely scary to think that five or ten years from now I'm going to be progressing through stages of Parkinson's disease," he says.

Bob has tried medication that helps most RBD sufferers (discussed later). And he and Lori have experimented with strategies to keep Bob sleeping and Lori safe, all to no avail.

Bob: "We've put a row of pillows in between us on the beds. We've slept in bigger beds."

Lori: "We've moved from a double bed to a queen-size bed. We went to twin beds."

"I kicked her right across the gap between us," says Bob.

"Every single night we say to each other, 'Have a good night, dear,'" says Lori. "And it's always the joke, because we don't. But, you know, at least you always hope."

SEXSOMNIA PLUS RBD

The Otts, on top of Tyson's sexsomnia, struggle with the same kind of RBD being endured in the Norman bedroom. Tyson's parasomnias also include sleep talking; not surprisingly, it's his wife he carries on conversations with while he's asleep.

"The other night, we're lying in bed," says Vanessa. "He sits up, looks over at me, and says: 'That's basically because I'm your boss.' And I said, 'Okay.' He acts out in his sleep probably at least three times a week. He's really getting worse about it. He's sitting up in bed and saying things to me, and trying to rip my clothes off and hold me down on the bed. I don't know if his eyes are open or not. It's so dark in our room that I really can't tell."

"I used to swing at her or kick at her, anything, while I was sleeping," says Tyson. "If she was trying to wake me up, I'd kick at her. I didn't even realize what I was doing."

Here's another odd feature: more than 80 percent of people with RBD are male. There are people who sleepwalk as children, continue to do so as adults, and are still at it when they're elderly. But often the onset of the behavior occurs after the age of fifty-five.

Vanessa and Tyson have two young children: Laney, three, and Sirus, eleven months.

"I love my kids to death," says Tyson, "and if I ever did anything to hurt them in any way, I would never forgive myself. It would kill me."

"I do worry that he could hurt our kids," says Vanessa. "I don't so much worry as long as I'm here, and we're all in the same house. But if I had to go out of town, or I was gone, then I would worry."

Why worry about Tyson attacking the kids in the night? Because the family co-sleeps in a king-size bed, lined up side by side. Vanessa sleeps between Tyson and the two children. Tyson has instructed his wife not to put the kids next to him while he's asleep.

It was the worry that Tyson could harm one of their children that prompted the couple to research his condition. They found a sexsomnia website—and suddenly realized that Tyson had something that could be diagnosed. "It sounded exactly like what we're going through," says Tyson. "I guess it's more reassuring that there's other people that are going through the same thing. But that still doesn't help me in my dealings with it. I'm not gonna say I'm a control freak. But I'm in control of most things in my life. I like it that way. But it's frightening to do something when you're so out of control that you don't know what the repercussions might be."

SWING SHIFT

Tyson works a swing shift: a week of twelve-hour days, then a week of twelve-hour nights. He thinks his work schedule has aggravated his parasomnias and added some of the additional problems that are common among shift workers: loss of memory, motor skills, and the ability to communicate.

"There's a lot of nights I get two hours, three hours of sleep," says Tyson. "I don't ever have any trouble falling asleep. I have trouble *staying* asleep. Sometimes I'll go to bed at ten o'clock and I'll wake up, get up at twelve-thirty. I won't be able to go back to sleep."

Tyson hasn't tried a sleep lab for a clearer diagnosis or medication that might help him. "I'm not so big on prescription drugs," he says. "Doctors are so quick to prescribe a lot of them nowadays. And, the long-term effects . . ." He lets it hang. But, he says, if it ever came to the point where he felt that he was a danger to his family, he would try just about anything. "I wouldn't think twice," he says.

TREATMENTS

There is help for people who suffer from REM behavior disorder. The first step is to go to a sleep lab for testing. REM behavior disorder, if that's your diagnosis, responds very well to long-acting benzodiazepine, a traditional prescription medication to promote sounder sleep. This medication, used on a nightly basis, is effective upward of 80 percent of the time.

"That's a pretty high success rate," says Dr. Cramer Bornemann of the University of Minnesota, who adds that he often sees quick results in his patients when they go on medication. "One of the fun things about doing sleep medicine is that you can come up with a diagnosis and get immediate impact. And it's not uncommon for patients or their partners to come back after the introduction of medication and say, 'We've had an incredible, miraculous turn of events.'"

Melatonin is another effective treatment for REM behavior disorder. It's something your body already produces—a hormone that helps regulate your sleep cycle. But melatonin as a medication has proven to be particularly effective for shift workers or people with jet lag—a reasonable alternative to the long-lasting sleep medications that are effective for RBD. "We have yet to understand the mechanism of it," says Bornemann. "But we're glad that we have an alternative."

Bornemann says a sleep lab study is crucial if you think you might have RBD. You want to make sure that what you have isn't obstructive sleep apnea. Do you snore a lot, hold your breath while you're asleep, and are you sleepy in the daytime? Those are all symptoms of apnea: problems breathing in the night. Awakening from a breath-holding spell when you have sleep apnea can actually trigger behaviors similar to RBD. Another thing a sleep study can rule out: epilepsy.

Sleep labs are fascinating places where doctors and technicians eavesdrop on your slumber. They glue a forest of electrodes to your scalp to monitor brain wave activity, more electrodes to get an EKG heart rhythm, and they monitor air flow, oxygen levels, and muscle movement.

Your whole night of sleep is there on their scopes. "We can tell when somebody's awake," says Bornemann, "when they're drifting to sleep. We can tell what degree of sleep they're in. We can look at breathing patterns and assess the degree of motor activity to see if it is consistent with RBD."

SLEEP DEPRIVATION

Who can tell if sleep disorders like sexsomnia and RBD will rise as our lives move more and more toward a twenty-four-hour day? Everyone in the field seems to agree that a good night's sleep is important for people with parasomnias—but it may be the hardest thing for them to get. Human beings have a hardwired, genetically programmed sleep requirement, and our mothers were right: most of us need eight hours of sleep a night. Of course, a lot of us aren't getting it.

"I can't tell you how many people say that they have conditioned themselves to only need five and a half hours of sleep," says Dr. Bornemann. "By and large, the statistics for that possibility are extremely low. More likely, they're running in a chronic sleep-deprived state."

Sleep deprivation only increases the likelihood of other parasomnias if you have a history of regular sleepwalking—one of the most common sleep disorders. As with many neurological conditions, doctors think there probably also is a genetic component involved.

So what's a "good night's sleep"? You don't just fall asleep and stay there—doctors talk about sleep in terms of stages or cycles, each one with a characteristic brain wave. Light sleep is typically stage one and stage two, and deep sleep is stages three and four. REM is traditionally seen as the deepest stage in sleep—when your body puts your major muscles out of commission and you dream.

Bornemann says the key is keeping those stages uninterrupted and intact. "We typically have anywhere from four to seven cycles in a complete eight-hour sleep period," he notes. "And REM accounts for about 25 percent of that sleep, with a majority of that REM associated with the last third of our sleep period."

With RBD and other parasomnias, "the body is now able to respond to some of the images or what we call dream mentation," says Bornemann. "REM behavior disorder tends to be a very sudden onset in dreams involving fear, fright, or flight. Either there is staving off an attacker, evading attack, or being involved in an attack. There's a very typical thematic component to RBD-related dreams. They're usually manifested in violent behaviors."

There have been criminal assault cases where RBD was used as a defense. But experts say that these odd REM sleep behaviors don't usually last long enough for a patient to harm someone, so usually RBD doesn't work as a legal defense.

So where is sexsomnia in all of this? Ironically, doctors say sexomnia is a "disorder of arousal"—and they mean arousal from sleep. It's not really associated with REM sleep; it happens when you're *not* dreaming—that can also be true with sleep talking, sleepwalking, sleep eating, and, in rare cases, sleeping while *driving an automobile*.

What struck us most about sexsomnia and RBD was how little of this we'd heard before. After all, everyone reading this book *sleeps*—but nobody gets a chance to observe their sleeping self. We'll spend a third of our life asleep, and (unless we go in for a sleep study) most of us won't have the vaguest idea of what goes on during our nights. That kind of ignorance is, medically speaking, bliss. People with parasomnias know all too well what they get up to once their heads hit the pillow.

7. PSEUDO SUICIDE

THEY WEREN'T DEPRESSED, ON DRUGS, OR PSYCHOTIC. THEY were two healthy young men who tried to kill themselves—or so it seemed.

In a bizarre instance of REM behavior disorder, Peter Polansky, an elite athlete who was ranked number one on Canada's junior tennis circuit, threw himself from the third-floor window of his hotel room in Mexico City. He had gone there in April 2006 to compete for the Davis Cup, and if he had died in the fall, his friends and family would have wondered why such a happy, successful young man had decided to take his own life.

It turned out that what looked like a suicide attempt happened in the middle of the night—when Peter was asleep. We bumped into his story when researching parasomnias—and it was one of the most dramatic ones out there.

A STRANGER IN THE ROOM

It was a fluke that his jump from the window didn't kill Peter—a hedge cushioned his fall. Hurtling into the hedge did, however, wake Peter up. He remembers sitting up, and realizing he was bleeding. "Help me, I'm dying," he remembers screaming. "I looked at my leg and it was cut open like a grapefruit. I couldn't believe it."

"He was basically bleeding to death," says Marlene Nobrega, a sports doctor who was traveling with Peter's Canadian tennis team. Her hotel phone had rung in the darkness, and a voice said, "You must come now, a guest has fallen." A second call came from the team captain, screaming, "Nobrega, it's Peter, come now." Seriously wounded but still conscious, Peter told Nobrega what he could remember. Someone in his hotel room was attacking him.

"I saw a black figure with a knife," Peter says. "I needed to get away." He went to the large window in his room, kicked it out, and threw himself through the shattered glass.

PETER WAS RUSHED to a nearby hospital. "He was about a millimeter away from severing the major artery to the leg," says Nobrega. "When someone loses that amount of blood, your biggest fear is that they will go into massive shock and the heart will stop."

Peter hung in there and pulled through.

Because he was part of a men's professional sports team, people assumed that somehow drugs or alcohol were involved in what had happened to Peter. There was speculation that the story of a stranger in his room was a cover for a wild party that had gone out of control.

The hospital did a toxicology screen for drugs and alcohol, which came back negative. His head coach, team captain, and a staff member from the Canadian embassy in Mexico City all convened and went through the hotel's videotapes and security log—no one had entered Peter's room the night of the fall. The only answer that fit was Peter's own explanation after reliving the "dark figure's" position in the room—that he had been dreaming and walking in his sleep.

After he was out of danger of dying, there was concern that Peter's leg would have to be amputated. He had lost a tremendous amount of blood and a nerve was severed. It seemed that if he did survive, he would never play tennis again. But after four hundred stitches and five weeks in a wheelchair, he worked his way back to a full recovery.

He's now back on the courts. "It will just be . . . what level can the coaches get him to," says Nobrega. "Athletes who go through very tough, traumatizing situations often come back better for it."

Peter knows how lucky he is. "I could have been on the tenth floor," he says. In which case he would have been a misunderstood footnote in men's tennis—the promising talent who killed himself. "Now when I travel or go anywhere, I get a room on the first floor with no windows. No nothing. In the basement."

SLEEPWALKING AND PSEUDO SUICIDE

Dr. Mark Mahowald, a neurologist and the medical director of the Minnesota Regional Sleep Disorders Center—and, incidentally, one of the world's experts on sleep disorders—says Peter was almost certainly sleepwalking the night of the accident: "Sleep terrors are characterized, often, by a sense of impending doom and a need to escape. And that's why people head toward windows. And if they're on the third or fourth floor, then they end up in real trouble."

As you'll remember from our chapter on sexsomnia, we normally pass through different stages when we sleep: wakefulness, when the brain is active but our muscles begin to relax; non-REM sleep, when our brain waves slow but our muscles are still active; and REM sleep, when our brains return to a level of activity that is pretty much the same as when we are awake, although we experience a complete paralysis of our voluntary muscles.

Mahowald says that these stages blending into each other can cause sleepwalking, a condition that is far more common than you might think, affecting about 4 percent of Americans. The cases where sleepwalking people have fatal accidents that are wrongly labeled suicides Dr. Mahowald calls "pseudo-suicides."

JAROD ALLGOOD

Becky Allgood is all too familiar with the term. In February of 1993, her world was shattered when police showed up at her door. Her twenty-one-year-old son, Jarod, dressed only in his boxer shorts, had sprinted through the freezing night and into the path of a truck on Highway 30 just south of Cedar Rapids, Iowa. He died instantly.

"The kids heard me scream, and then I got sick," says Becky. "Then I started asking questions." Her mother's intuition: this just didn't make sense.

The next morning, police showed up at Jarod's apartment to interview his roommate and best friend, Jeff Harris.

"I was in total shock," Harris recalls, when the police showed him a photo of Jarod's face taken in the morgue. "He didn't have any enemies, so I didn't think it was foul play. He did the normal college kid drinking thing, but not that week. No drugs."

The night of the incident, Jeff and Jarod had come back to their apartment after a weekend in Manchester, going to the movies and visiting their girlfriends. Jarod went to bed at midnight, saying he was tired. He was asleep when Jeff went to bed two hours later.

Jeff was surprised when the police started asking questions that made it seem as though Jarod might have committed suicide.

"All of a sudden, they were asking me if he had been depressed or anything," Jeff says. "Jarod wasn't a depressed kid."

A RECURRING DREAM

If he didn't want to kill himself, what could possibly have compelled Jarod to wander out in his boxers, with snow on the ground, across deserted sidewalks, down a road, and finally, out onto a four-lane highway? The quarter-mile trip made no sense to Becky. She asked Jeff to give her all the details that might explain her son's death. As mother and best friend talked, a curious detail emerged. Jeff mentioned that Jarod had had a recurring dream: he was running a race with a man from Bertram, which was down the road from their apartment.

"He was sleepwalking!" Becky blurted out as she remembered that Jarod had had instances of odd sleeping behavior as a child.

That made sense to Jeff. He'd seen Jarod sleepwalk. One night, Jarod, with eyes wide open, had walked out of his bedroom wearing only his boxer shorts. "Too dark in here," he said. He opened the curtains in the room, turned on the lights, and then went back into his bedroom. When Jeff opened his bedroom door, Jarod was fast asleep. The next morning, Jarod had absolutely no recollection of it. The two friends were puzzled—not alarmed.

But could Jarod possibly have run, sleeping, for a quarter mile, nearly naked and barefoot on a snowy winter night, and not woken up?

Dr. Mahowald says that is well within the range of possibility. "There have been instances where people have actually shot themselves in the leg while sleepwalking," he says. "And it wasn't until the sleepwalking was over that they realized that they had injured themselves. So pain is generally not perceived during sleep."

CAUSE OF DEATH

Although Mahowald believed Jarod's behavior that night was consistent with sleepwalking, local authorities were skeptical. There were reports around town that Jarod had committed suicide. The death certificate listed the cause of death as "Undetermined."

"I said no!" Becky recalls. "It needs to say, 'Hit by a truck while sleepwalking.' You need to say why he died."

Mahowald helped her make her case. "The primary determinant of whether someone is going be a sleepwalker or not is a positive family history," Mahowald says.

"All my kids walk in their sleep," says Becky. "Jarod had night terrors. He never woke up; he just would scream."

Becky says she never thought she would lose a child to what seemed a strange but generally harmless family trait.

Jarod's sleep history, recurring dream, and his mother's persistence eventually convinced Iowa's chief medical examiner to change Jarod's official cause of death to "Sleepwalking."

Becky says: "I believe that it's the first death certificate that has ever, in this state, even acknowledged sleep disorders in any way."

Experts are left to wonder: how many other sleepwalking deaths have been mistakenly labeled suicide?

8. MAD AS A HATTER

SOME OF THE MOST BAFFLING CASES CAN HAPPEN TO THE MOST savvy patients. Sometimes the patient is a doctor—puzzling through the symptoms right along with her colleagues. Such was the case of Hayley Rintel, a twenty-seven-year-old medical resident at Christiana Care Hospital in Newark, Delaware, who knew something was very wrong.

In September 2005, Hayley found herself in the emergency room of her own hospital—not looking at X-rays or starting someone's IV, but lying on a gurney in the middle of the night. She was clearly sick—but she had absolutely no idea what the problem was. And her friends, her fellow doctors, were just as confused.

A NORMAL DAY

It had been a normal day for Hayley—which meant she was caring for newborn babies in the hospital's neonatal intensive care unit. She left work at about 4:30 P.M., hit the gym for her usual cardio workout, and then had what she remembers as a delicious dinner at home with her then-fiancé, Sean Queller.

They were both careful about eating healthy food—Sean was a great gardener and grew a lot of their vegetables. Dinner was the last normal thing about that night.

"I was upstairs reading in my bed, feeling a little bit lightheaded," Hayley says. "I couldn't get a deep breath in. I wasn't seeing as clearly as I thought I should. I felt very thirsty. My arms were heavy. My legs were very heavy. I couldn't sit up. Something was wrong."

It was worse when she tried to explain it to Sean. Hayley's speech was garbled; she seemed increasingly incoherent, consumed by anxiety. She felt as though she was on fire, but she couldn't get up to go to the bathroom and get a drink. That's when she decided to go to the ER. Sean had to dress her and carry her downstairs to the car. It was shortly after midnight when the couple entered the emergency room of Christiana. Dr. Jonathan McGhee, a colleague and osteopath, recognized Hayley right away.

"Hayley and I started as interns together," McGhee says. "It was a surprise to see her in the ER that night."

McGhee discovered that Hayley's heart rate was up, in the one-fifties, and her respiratory rate was higher than it should have been. Hayley responded incoherently to the questions of the nurses and physicians who examined her. "They'd ask her questions, and she had no clue what they were saying," Sean recalls. "She was saying things that didn't make any sense."

"I couldn't understand why people couldn't understand me," Hayley says. "I thought I was speaking clear as day. They took my blood pressure. I remember looking at the blood pressure and saying, 'Wow, that patient's blood pressure is very high.' It took me a little bit to realize that it was *me*!"

There were periods when Hayley was lucid—then she would spout gibberish again. McGhee says: "She was talking about things that she was supposed to be doing as a resident upstairs when, obviously, she was a patient in the emergency department. She alluded to people that weren't in the room."

At one point, Hayley donned examination gloves and talked about doing a rectal exam on a patient in another room.

"The nurses had fun with that," McGhee recalls. "It made for quite a conversation."

"ALL THE WORST THINGS"

As a doctor, Hayley knew all the potentially deadly diseases that could be responsible for the symptoms she was experiencing. She ran through them in her head: might she be having a stroke? "I've been on the other side, knowing [which diseases] could actually present in that manner," Hayley says. "I definitely was thinking [of] all the worst things." She felt things crawling on her. She realized she was hallucinating and not making sense.

After taking a quick medical history, McGhee asked Hayley if she was getting enough sleep. Perhaps she was anxious because she was tired and overworked? He thought perhaps her symptoms might be caused by some sort of psychotic break.

"At the time," Hayley recalls, "I was taking [medication] for depression. And they thought: 'Maybe the pressure's getting to her and she snapped.' I *was* working long hours in the neonatal ICU, which is definitely a difficult place to be. But I was happy. I had just moved into a new home. I was engaged.

I was planning a big wedding. I wasn't anxious about my life at that point."

McGhee thought Hayley might be having an adverse reaction to her medication for depression. Then he thought that she might have been exposed to a toxin. "I asked her what she had had for dinner," McGhee says. "She told me turkey burgers, roasted vegetables, and a salad of lettuce from their garden. We talked about [the toxicity of] some organic pesticides that you can spray on the lettuce. We use the word 'toxidrome' to describe a set of symptoms that goes along with having ingested a particular class of drugs. They present with a fast heart rate, dry mouth, breathing a little bit faster than you might normally breathe. There's a big subset of young adults who use drugs recreationally. Our urine tox screen tests for amphetamines, barbiturates, cocaine, marijuana."

None of those were present in Hayley's blood. An MRI was negative as well, for both stroke and a brain tumor—so it wasn't a physical lump in her brain that was causing Hayley's symptoms. A CAT scan of Hayley's chest, to rule out clots in her lungs that could have caused her shortness of breath, also came back normal.

"We thought about her thyroid being out of whack," says McGhee. "But the test indicated that she had an *under*active thyroid, which didn't fit with her high heart rate. The [test results] were vague and not really helpful. We didn't have a good grasp on what was going on and didn't feel safe enough to send her home."

ADMITTED FOR OBSERVATION

During this long night of seemingly endless and inconclusive tests, Sean was beside himself. It didn't make him feel any better when the doctors admitted that they might not be able to make a diagnosis.

"We decided to go ahead and admit her to the hospital for a period of observation," says McGhee.

Although Hayley's blood pressure was still high, by seven or eight o'clock in the morning she was able to speak clearly, and she knew where she was. She could converse, but her body felt strange.

"I didn't feel like myself," she says. "I felt very tired, almost like I had just played a full game of soccer. I was so fatigued. Every time I went to the bathroom or walked out to tell the nurse something, my cardiac alarm would go off because my heart rate would just go right through the roof. It would make me short of breath to walk fifteen feet. I was very wobbly, sort of seasick."

After a few days in the hospital, Hayley couldn't wait to get home. She was happy there as a doctor, but not as a patient. "I definitely now have an appreciation for how people feel when they're in the hospital," she says. "It's not fun. Even though I love Christiana and the people are great, I couldn't wait to leave."

Christiana Care Hospital finally discharged Hayley after four days. Diagnosis? Unknown. They told her that they were confident that nothing terrible was happening to her—after all, all her tests were normal. But Hayley was worried: Whatever it was, would it come back? Was there some hidden problem in her body that medical tests just couldn't locate?

MAD AS A HATTER

After her release, Hayley rested. She had follow-up examinations with a cardiologist and a neurologist. Her heart rate continued to be elevated for a week and a half after she was discharged. Her mother and younger sister took care of her while Sean was away at work. All the while, the young doctor chewed over her symptoms, her tests—and got no closer to an answer.

That is, until she went outside.

The pieces in the puzzle of Hayley's medical mystery fell into place when she decided to tend her garden. Ordered by her doctors and family to rest, she hadn't been outside for days. But this day "I felt good enough to go out and water the garden," Hayley says. "There was a plant with beautiful white flowers on it growing right in the middle of our lettuce patch."

Hayley says she immediately knew that the plant had to be responsible for what had happened to her. She dug one up and put it in a bag. Her mother drove her to the local nursery. Hayley began to remove the plant from the bag to show it to the woman who worked there. But the woman jumped, and told Hayley not to touch the plant, that it was toxic and if it got into her skin she could go crazy. Hayley told the woman that she had just gotten out of the hospital. "I think I ate some of it!" she remembers saying. The woman was astonished that Hayley was still around to tell the tale.

The lovely white flower Hayley had found goes by a number of names: jimsonweed, locoweed, and angel's trumpet. Jimsonweed rang a bell for Hayley. In medical school, she had learned the mnemonic—"red as a beet, dry as a bone, hot as a hare, blind as a bat, mad as a hatter"—a constellation of symptoms that spelled jimsonweed poisoning.

"If I wasn't in the medical field," Hayley says, "it wouldn't have clicked right away. When I got home, and saw this weed growing in my garden, I probably would have picked it and thrown it out. But in my mind-set I *had* to find out what was wrong with me. I needed to know because I didn't want to be worried that I'm going to land in the hospital again. As soon as I saw that plant, I knew right away. Every time I see a new patient, I ask them about their diet, new food exposures, and travel history."

Such a simple explanation after so many tests—in the haystack that is all of our body's systems and functions, the "needle" of what's wrong is often tremendously hard to spy.

Jimsonweed crops up in different places. It is well known to shamans—and people who want to get high—for its hallucinogenic properties. Berton Roueché, in his book *The Medical Detectives*, writes that Jimsonweed (*Datura*) gives off a fetid smell. Its fruit, or seed pod, is barbed with thorns, like a chestnut bur. The poisonous flowers, milky white and sometimes streaked with purple, are trumpet-shaped and beautiful. The plant often reaches a height of six feet—livestock are generally repelled by the smell, but hungry animals have been known to eat it. Jimson seeds and leaves are sometimes accidentally harvested with hay, poisoning livestock.

Hayley says there are medicines to treat "anticholinergic toxidrome," which is the kind of poisoning Jimsonweed produces, but you have to be sure that it is the poison you're dealing with. Otherwise the "cure" can have side effects that will harm someone who has another syndrome.

"In retrospect, I wasn't sick enough to warrant using the medication," says Hayley (now Dr. Queller and married to Sean). "But I certainly fit the mnemonic." Hayley says if she or her colleagues had thought of Jimsonweed's five symptoms, it would have made her life a whole lot easier. She certainly felt "mad as a hatter" that night in the emergency room!

And yes, as soon as she returned home from the nursery, Hayley—very carefully, wearing gloves—pulled the rest of the Jimsonweed from her vegetable patch and got rid of it. I guess the moral of this story is to keep a sharp eye on your own garden—you never know what might be growing there.

9. LLAMAS?

ADMITTEDLY, HER ILLNESS WAS FASCINATING, BUT IT WAS THE llamas that got us interested. Diana Wyman, who lives in Cornish Flat, New Hampshire, and raises llamas, had become tremendously ill. Her doctors were struggling to find out why. After all, she had always been healthy, even baking her own bread and eating organic food. Was there a parasite that moved from llama to human? A strange llama disease that could be transmitted?

Diana first landed at her family doctor's office with a straightforward problem: an ear infection that was causing her to lose her hearing. The doctor prescribed antibiotics. But as is occasionally the case, the pills upset Diana's stomach. She started losing weight: ten pounds in two weeks. Worse, she seemed generally unwell—her husband, Curtis, a mechanic, says that she was sleeping eighteen hours a day. Her son was worried, too.

"I was exhausted," says Diana. "I had a rash but I wasn't sure what it was. My knees started burning."

"She had a little bit of blood when she brushed her teeth," says Curtis. "She was sick. But Diana is a stubborn Armenian!"

"I am stubborn," Diana admits.

So stubborn in fact that even with her exhaustion and the other symptoms, she kept up with her chores, feeding the llamas. She wouldn't go back to the doctor, either, and insisted on going about her life as usual, bruised and in pain, when she was able to hobble out of bed. "It was just like a sprained ankle, pulled muscle, minor cramp," says Diana. "Thought I could walk it out. But it kept getting a little bit worse. I was just pushing. Until I couldn't. I got up to go to the bathroom, took two steps, and couldn't take any more. It hurt too bad."

This time her husband wouldn't take no for an answer. He wrapped Diana in a blanket and carried his wife to the car and back to the doctor. Diana remembers little of the journey. "I know I felt awful," she says. "I wanted to just curl up in the fetal position." Her primary physician sent her to the emergency ward.

In the emergency ward, Dr. Osei Bonsu got her case. "I immediately concluded that this lady might have cancer," he says. "She came in with leg pain, could not walk. Her feet and legs were swollen, and [she] had lost some weight. Felt weak, and you know, had rashes on her legs and feet."

When he took her family history, he found out she had been a smoker, which was a concern. Even in those who've quit there's an elevated risk of cancer.

"If you have cancer that's spread all over, to your spine, to your liver, and in your blood vessels, those vessels could get blocked and you could get swelling," Bonsu says.

Curtis mentioned that the couple raised llamas. Perhaps, Bonsu thought, she had picked up some kind of exotic disease from the animals. He also thought about vasculitis, a condition where your blood vessels are damaged, inflamed—especially the arteries—and which produces some of the symptoms Diana had been experiencing, especially her weakness and general malaise. It can be quite serious.

The doctors ordered tests—a CAT scan and an ultrasound of her legs and abdomen to look for tumors, clots, or anything else that might be interfering with her circulation. To say the Wymans were alarmed would be a vast understatement. Doctors weren't talking about her simple ear infection anymore—all the tests they conducted were for potentially life-threatening illnesses.

But even those tests didn't seem to help—all of them came back negative. The doctors could shed absolutely no light on Diana's strange bundle of symptoms.

At this point, Dr. Jennifer Quinn, a resident in internal medicine, remembers looking at Diana, a tiny woman. Diana's legs were so swollen that they looked as though they belonged to somebody else. Quinn was as bewildered as the rest.

"Some people *say*, 'I can't walk,'" says Quinn. "But they're [actually] walking with pain. She really *couldn't* walk at all! She had all this horrible bruising. Plus she had all these little sub-skin hemorrhages everywhere. I've never seen all of that together in one person."

Blood tests were ordered. "They were drawing blood out of her like a sieve," says Curtis.

Again, they waited for test results. But once again the blood work didn't turn up anything. Diana's blood count was normal. She was a little low on her red blood cells, but that isn't unusual for someone who is pre-menopausal.

The doctors were frustrated.

"As a physician, your tests are done to confirm what you suspect the diagnosis is," says Quinn. "It was really disturbing that I didn't have a good sense other than some vague notion of, you know, llamas, vasculitis, hepatitis maybe . . ."

There was concern that the swelling in Diana's legs was going to compromise her circulation—if the blood can't get to your extremities, they can die off. She could lose toes, even a foot. And if she had a clot in the veins of her legs, Quinn says, that "could be pretty serious, because those clots can embolize, they can migrate into the lungs and can actually ultimately be fatal."

The doctors began to consider calling in a surgeon to make incisions to relieve some of that swelling. The thought of surgery and the expanding bevy of doctors and their uncertainty frightened Diana and Curtis. "I'm a very good mechanic and I can take apart a million-dollar machine," says Curtis. "But I can't take a person apart." He said he felt "helpless, very helpless."

"I was scared," says Diana. "I didn't want to have an operation."

IN MEDICINE, one of your best weapons against disease is often consultation—if you can't figure out what's going on, you call in all the medical minds you can find. A senior internist—Dr. Jonathan Ross, the attending physician at the hospital—was brought in to look at Diana's case. "The red spots that I expected to see as consistent with vasculitis looked very different," Ross recalls. He asked what turned out to be the key question. "I began to ask a couple of questions about her diet. . . ."

What he found was startling. Diana's normal diet was extremely restricted. ("I can name the foods she eats on five fingers," her husband says.) During her course of antibiotics, when her stomach was upset, her food choice had narrowed even more. She had been living, almost exclusively, on peanut butter!

"My day just wasn't right without it," says Diana.

The next morning, the hospital staff met, and Dr. Ross made a diagnosis that floored his colleagues. "I think she has scurvy," Ross said.

"We all basically looked at each other and were, like, in shock," says Bonsu.

"You've got to be kidding," Quinn remembers blurting out. "Somebody even went, 'Yar!'"

Scurvy—a syndrome caused by vitamin C deficiency—just doesn't happen very much anymore. Hippocrates, the ancient Greek doctor, described it, but you've probably only heard of it as a problem that sea voyagers would get in previous centuries, because of their diet of hardtack and rum. But vitamin C is something everybody needs, and you have to get it from your diet. It's used internally to construct strong collagen tissues—and those are found in blood vessels, skin, joints, muscles, and your heart.

The cure? Getting some vitamin C. In 1536 the French explorer Jacques Cartier, sailing Canada's St. Lawrence River, used the local natives' knowledge to save his men from scurvy. They taught him to boil the needles of the arbor vitae tree (eastern white cedar) to make a tea that was later shown to contain 50 mg of vitamin C per 100 grams. It was a Scottish surgeon in the British Royal Navy, James Lind, who first proved scurvy could be treated with citrus fruit, in experiments he described in his 1753 book, *A Treatise of the Scurvy*. Sailors used to hoard citrus fruit on board to try to prevent it.

In fact, the limes the British Royal Navy brought aboard their ships to prevent scurvy are why the British were nicknamed "limeys."

Back to Diana: if scurvy is untreated it is invariably fatal—but once it's diagnosed, it is easily cured.

"They dumped two IVs of vitamin C into Diana," says Curtis. "And within twelve hours, it started to make a big difference."

"Within forty-eight hours, I was getting my feet back," says Diana.

Today, Diana is fine, making sure she eats more than just peanut butter. She says she's learned—the hard way—the importance of proper nutrition.

"I've got to take care of myself," she says. After all, she has llamas to worry about.

10. AFTER THE HONEYMOON

"I HAD JUST GOTTEN MARRIED TO THE MAN OF MY DREAMS AND had a beautiful wedding and we were living in New York City, and I was very excited to get on with the new phase in my life." So says twenty-five-year-old Suzanne. After the wedding, she and her husband, a high school coach, went on a Caribbean honeymoon and then returned to the Big Apple, ready to begin their life together.

They had no idea what was in store for them. Soon after they returned, Suzanne awoke in the middle of the night with a sharp pain in her chest. She felt as though she was having a heart attack, or had been stabbed. She sat up and turned to her sleeping husband, but speaking—even breathing—was unbearably painful. He calmed her down, and the pain subsided.

"I felt a little foolish about making such a big deal over something that had come out of nowhere and gone just as quickly," says Suzanne. "I've been very healthy my whole life. To have such an extreme pain was frightening."

The couple decided to wait until morning to seek medical help.

The next day, Suzanne's doctor, though obviously concerned, was reassuring as well. Healthy, Caucasian, young—women like this are at just about the lowest risk for heart attacks, he told her. The sharp pain she had experienced could have been caused by acid reflux—possibly stress from her recent wedding.

To be on the safe side, he sent Suzanne for an EKG and X-rays. He was stunned, and so was Suzanne, at the result: an obvious abnormality in the lungs. This healthy, happy young woman clearly had some serious medical issue, and needed a CAT scan as soon as possible.

AN AMBIGUOUS ABNORMALITY

Sometimes fate hands you a lucky card. Suzanne's godmother, Dr. Maureen Zakowski, is a specialist at Memorial Sloan-Kettering Cancer Center. As a senior attending pathologist, she diagnoses tissue samples and solves medical mysteries for a living. Her specialty: the lungs. Suzanne called her godmother in a panic and, with X-ray films in hand, went to Zakowski's apartment.

When Zakowski saw the film, she gasped. It clearly showed a density, a lesion, some sort of abnormality—in *both* lungs. Zakowski wanted a radiologist to have a look at the films as quickly as possible.

"I've literally known her since before she was born," Zakowski says of Suzanne. "I actually did the over-the-counter pregnancy test for her mom. I've been to her graduations and her wedding. I gave the bridal shower. She's lovely, intelligent, beautiful. She's totally healthy, active, athletic. Suzanne is like a combination of my little sister and daughter. I was very frightened when I saw the chest film. I didn't want Suzanne to know how frightened I was."

Zakowski thought her goddaughter might have lung cancer, lymphoma, or Hodgkin's disease, although she hoped the lesions she saw on the film indicated something as simple and straightforward as pneumonia.

By the time Suzanne had the CAT scan, she was in tremendous discomfort. She could barely breathe, walk up stairs, swallow, or cough. She took the slides immediately to Sloan-Kettering, where Zakowski showed them to Dr. Michelle Ginsberg, a radiologist.

"The findings were so evident that you could have seen them from across the room," says Ginsberg.

Zakowski and Ginsberg sat down with Suzanne in Ginsberg's office.

"They told me they were going to sort of talk out loud and rule things out," says Suzanne. "They threw out a lot of words. They pointed at the images and said okay, this looks like cancer, but over here, this doesn't."

The doctors had three possible diagnoses: pneumonia, an allergic reaction, or cancer. Suzanne had chest pain and a cough but no fever or night sweats. The doctors wondered if there was something that could have triggered an allergic reaction. Had Suzanne been exposed to any new pets? Drugs?

"Pneumonia can look like and mimic lung cancer or lymphoma," says Ginsberg. "It's hard to tell from the CAT scan. You really need a tissue diagnosis."

As the doctors conferred, Suzanne felt that at least she knew there was a reason for the pain she had been feeling—she'd wondered about the stress of the wedding and feared her symptoms might be "all in her head."

"The CAT scan confirmed that I was, indeed, in tremendous pain, which was nice to hear from a doctor," she says.

"The lesions had adhered to the pleura, which is the lining of your lung, which is like a whole bundle of raw nerves."

THE TEAM GETS GOING

Every disease at Sloan-Kettering gets a disease management team, which means that experts in all aspects of a disease work together. Zakowski and Ginsberg worked on a daily basis with lung surgeons, lung oncologists, and lung radiation oncologists. They were part of the lung team.

On Fridays, the lung team met to discuss patients. That Friday, Zakowski grabbed a couple of people at the end of the meeting and told them that they had to have a look at Suzanne's scans and examine her.

"Clear your schedule," Zakowski remembers saying. "If she's going to have surgery, it has to be next week. They let me pull rank. We scheduled her to be seen by a medical doctor and a thoracic surgeon, who would be the person to operate should [that] be indicated. And I chose a thoracic surgeon who was very approachable and calm and confident."

BRONCHOSCOPY

Suzanne was scheduled for a bronchoscopy, during which a flexible tube with a scope would be inserted into her lungs so that the doctors could have a look and take tissue samples. It's an uncomfortable procedure, but a much cheaper, faster, safer way to get a diagnosis than doing exploratory surgery.

Zakowski laughs when she recalls Suzanne's pre-op encounter with a handsome medic.

"When she was about to get her bronchoscopy done," says Zakowski, "she thought there was a particularly cute fellow who was involved in the procedure, and she was determined to get his name or his e-mail address for her girlfriend. And she kept saying, 'Not me, not me, I'm just married. This is for my girlfriend.' She went into her sedation, saying, 'Please, please, just give me your e-mail!' She's always looking out for her girlfriends. But he wouldn't budge."

Unfortunately, the doctors couldn't remove enough of the tissue during the bronchoscopy for the biopsy to be conclusive. They strongly suspected, however, that Suzanne had some type of cancer, and they decided to schedule her for full surgery to remove a piece of her right lung.

Zakowski knew that both of Suzanne's parents were smokers. And her father had had a recent lung lesion, which had been diagnosed by Ginsberg. "It was benign, nothing to worry about," Zakowski says. "But the whole experience of anything in the lung in her family was utter panic for Suzanne. She was already imagining her funeral."

SURGERY

Zakowski says that Suzanne's fears were well founded. The doctors knew that if it was cancer it was incurable. There were simply too many lesions in both lungs.

During the surgery, Zakowski and Ginsberg were standing by in what is called the "frozen section" of the pathology department, where tissue samples from the operating room are examined. During this process, the patient remains under anesthesia and the surgeon is waiting in the wings for a diagnosis. His next move depends on what the tissue sample indicates. Should he remove the lung, if it's a malignancy, or end the procedure and close the chest back up?

As Zakowski sliced the tissue, her relief was clear. The sample didn't look like cancer at all. In fact, Zakowski was sure, given the appearance of the tissue sample, that what she had was an inflammatory condition—a reaction to something that was irritating her goddaughter's lungs in a very serious way.

"My job is to diagnose lung cancer," Zakowski says. "I have many years of experience. I'm supposed to know what cancer looks like, and I knew this was not cancer. I was so grateful and happy."

Suzanne remembers being woken up by her surgeon, who told her that she didn't have cancer. Great. But they didn't know what she *did* have.

"I was so relieved," says Suzanne. "At the same time, it was very painful to breathe after surgery. Recovering from surgery is its own experience. They had severed nerves to go into my rib cage. I stayed in the hospital for about three more days to do respiratory treatments, to get my breathing back. But I still had all these undiagnosed lesions in my lungs."

A DIAGNOSIS

After sifting through the evidence, Zakowski finally realized that Suzanne might have something completely unexpected: eosinophilic pneumonia, an infection that was infiltrating and destroying her healthy lung tissue. The cause: an adverse reaction to a drug.

"What are you taking, Suzanne?" Zakowski asked. The implication was that her godmother was accusing Suzanne of taking illicit drugs.

"All I'm taking are birth control pills and [an] antibiotic," Suzanne replied.

Zakowski told Suzanne to immediately discontinue all medications. The lesions could be a rare side effect—an inflammatory allergic response to what Suzanne had thought was a harmless drug to prevent, of all things, acne.

"I had been taking an antibiotic . . . leading up to my wedding, to prevent [acne] outbreaks," says Suzanne. "Once I told them I had been on this antibiotic, a lightbulb went off. This antibiotic has been associated with this type of pneumonia in the past. It was exactly what had caused the lesions."

Suzanne was shocked that such a seemingly innocuous medication could have caused such an adverse reaction. As soon as she stopped taking it, she began to improve.

"Any drug can do *anything* in the right environment," says Zakowski. "And this fairly innocent drug had caused a horrific lung response that could eventually have killed her."

Suzanne says she was taking the drug because a wedding planning calendar told all brides to consult a dermatologist—and the dermatologist's recommendation was to go on the antibiotic to make sure she didn't break out on her big day.

"I took it without question and I definitely regret doing that," Suzanne says. "I often forgot to take it. I had taken it casually after the wedding because I was told not to stop antibiotics abruptly, to finish the course."

And sure, her wedding pictures look great. But if she hadn't found the cause of her medical mystery, her honeymoon would have probably been the end of her marriage, and of her.

"I certainly don't think that her prescribing physician was at fault," says Zakowski. "It was a very uncommon side effect."

"I think my experience was a perfect example of a widely held belief in our culture that there's a cure-all pill for everything," says Suzanne. "My experience definitely proves that that's not true. We live in a culture where people are overmedicated and don't ask enough questions. We all need to be responsible for what we put into our bodies. I can't take antibiotics ever again. And I had a large piece of my lung removed. I put my family through the wringer. It was a very difficult experience, and the only good that will come from this is to try to get the word out."

"Why do you have to take antibiotics because you're going to get married?" Zakowski asks. "There's kind of an industry out there. And I think she fell victim to that industry image. She's a beautiful girl; she didn't need to do that."

Suzanne says Zakowski saved her life: "I feel incredibly lucky that she made it her mission to get to the bottom of this as quickly as possible."

Their relationship had always been about more than just wedding showers and birthday gifts. But after her near death, the relationship has become even more special. As Suzanne now puts it, "Maureen is absolutely my fairy godmother."

11. BIONIC WOMAN

THE FEELING OF COOL WATER ON YOUR HAND, THE TOUCH OF A soft blanket on your fingertips. Would you be able to feel them if your hand was no longer there? Before you answer, read Claudia's story. If you're like the *Medical Mysteries* producers, it will take your mind a moment to wrap itself around the concept.

Claudia Mitchell is a college student and former Marine who gives a whole new meaning to the term touchy-feely—the feelings in *her* hand are pretty extraordinary. Because she gets them when you touch her chest. You read that right. Touch her chest, and she'll feel it in her hand—a hand that *isn't there*. It's confusing, but read on. That's just part of the mystery and the miracle of the world's first "bionic woman."

When Claudia lost her left arm in a motorcycle accident, she was given the standard prosthesis. You strap on an artificial arm and use the muscles of your shoulder to push the rigid arm into different positions. But Claudia was uncomfortable with it; it was hard to use, and she ended up not wearing it much. She was more than ready to volunteer for the experimental surgery that would change her life.

The surgical team, led by Dr. Todd Kuiken of the Rehabilitation Institute of Chicago, tried an unexpected tack. They took the severed, dormant nerves in Claudia's shoulder, nerves that had controlled the movement of her arm, and put them *under* the muscle in her chest. They wanted the implanted nerves to reawaken and control a new type of computer-driven robotic arm.

Kuiken explains how this new type of human-machine melding works, activated by the muscles of Claudia's chest: "When the muscle contracts, it lets these little bits of electricity out. We have tiny antennas built into the part that sits on her chest, and they pick up those electrical signals. We then have a computer that decodes those signals and tells the artificial arm what to do." What they've done seems like a miracle—Claudia controls her robotic arm the same way you control *your* arm: with her thoughts.

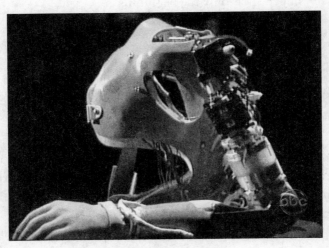

Claudia's new arm.

EUREKA!

Now she can just think, "Move your arm," and her arm does what she commands. "All I have to think is that I want my hand to open, and that muscle automatically responds," says Claudia. "I think, 'Open and close my hand,' and it does."

Claudia had mourned the end of what we all take for granted, a two-armed life. It included the ability, for instance, to open a jar or put on makeup. But since her nerves were reawakened, it's constant discovery.

"I have what I call my 'eureka' moments," she says. "My stunned, just amazing, I-can't-believe-I-just-did-that moments! Being able to fold my shirt while I'm standing up. Being able to hold my squash while I cut it up into my pan."

Claudia was delighted with her newfound abilities and the way her new prosthesis responded to the messages from her brain. But this was only the beginning.

A ROBOT THAT FEELS

While Claudia was on the operating table, the surgeons went deep under the muscles in her shoulder to see exactly where her remaining, healthy nerves were located and where they went. Then they carefully isolated those nerves that had carried signals to her arm—not just "motor signals," how the arm got its instructions to move, but "sensory signals"—the signals that gave her arm *feeling*.

Then they moved some of the nerves in her chest muscles over—to put the arm nerves next to them. "We got them out of the way and let the new nerves grow into those muscles [in her chest]," says Kuiken. "Finally, we cut a little nerve just over her collarbone that provides sensation for a patch about the size of a softball on her chest and sewed her up."

When Claudia came out of the anesthesia, the place near her collarbone where nerves had been cut was numb, completely devoid of sensation. But over the next few months, things began to happen.

"The hand motor nerves grew into these [chest] muscles, and she started to get little twitches when she thought about closing her hand or bending the elbow," said Kuiken. "And as the weeks went on, they got stronger and stronger. This little spot that had gone numb also started to regain sensation. But it was the sensation *of her hand*. So if you touched Claudia here," Kuiken indicates a spot on his chest, "she feels her thumb. You touch [another spot] and she can feel a finger."

Claudia is able to experience a variety of sensations in what feels like her hand, the hand that was amputated. Here's the part that takes a moment to understand: she doesn't feel "her hand" in her prosthetic robot hand, she feels it on her chest. That's where surgeons redirected the nerves that used to connect her brain to the skin of her hand.

Claudia had been forewarned by Kuikan that she might begin to experience sensation in her missing limb, but it took some months after the surgery for the new connections to begin to work. Claudia recalls her excitement when she first became fully aware of what was happening: "I wasn't sure what to expect, but was expecting something. So I'm standing in the shower. I had hot water on me. And all of a sudden, I could feel hot water in my hand. And not this one," she says, pointing to the prosthetic. She could feel it in the hand that was no longer there. "I was so excited. I hurried up and I toweled off. I called up Chicago and told the doctors: It's working. It's working! I can feel my hand in my chest! *I felt hot water!*"

Spooky—Claudia feels these sensations in her missing hand. And she spends a lot of time explaining it to people. Before the amputation, "I had a nerve that let me know what I was feeling in my hand," she says. "Well, they took that nerve and put it under skin on my chest. So I have an area on my chest that, when it's touched, it feels like something's touching my hand."

And now when hot water runs over that patch of skin on her chest, Claudia "feels" it in her missing hand.

The range of sensations amazes both Claudia and her medical team. "When someone touches my chest, I can feel different locations in my hand," she says. "I can discriminate whether it's my pinkie or my index finger or my thumb. And I can feel different sensations, hot and cold, and if someone is putting pressure on it or if it's just a light touch."

ROBUST PATHWAYS

Kuiken says that Claudia was lucky. Her brain was still sending strong signals to her amputated limb. "The fact is that Claudia's brain was able to immediately send out these commands to control her missing arm," said Kuiken. "And she was immediately, once the nerves were connected, able to feel her missing hand. So those pathways in the brain were very robust. They endured."

Kuiken explained that following an amputation, the part of the brain that responds to signals from the amputated limb will shrink, but that other sections will take over that function. "We didn't really know what would happen on the brain level," he says. "We assumed that it would work, but we didn't know how the brain might change."

The strength of Claudia's brain signals made Kuiken believe they might be able to successfully re-map both the motor and sensory nerves of her severed arm to that area of skin on her chest, and to the healthy muscle tissue under her breasts. This was groundbreaking.

BIONIC BEGINNINGS

Kuiken had come close to this result before, more or less by accident.

"On our first patient, Jesse Sullivan, we did the nerve transfers into muscle," says Kuiken. "My goal was to let him operate a prosthetic arm better. But then, after about six months, one of the team was rubbing some alcohol on his chest as we got ready to do an experiment, and he started blowing on it. And he says, 'Oooh, that's cold in my hand.' Sensation started to grow into his chest skin so that Jesse, when you pressed him in different places, felt different parts of his hand. That was a complete surprise to us. I had to think about what it meant. What I could do with it. And the more we thought about it, the more excited we got."

Kuiken knew he'd found "a portal into the nervous system to provide sensation feedback."

Then he met Claudia.

"Claudia was the first person whose skin we purposely reinnervated with her hand sensation nerves," Kuiken says.

"Reinnervation" is the term used when surgeons restore function to tissue—usually muscle tissue—by giving it a new nerve supply, usually by grafting.

What Kuiken did with Claudia went quite a bit further, however. Remember, there are two different kinds of nerves—motor nerves that tell the muscles what to do and sensation nerves that take information from your skin and feed it back up to the brain.

The network of nerves Dr. Kuiken created in Claudia's chest is not simple. It's not as if they placed specific nerves for specific functions or sensations in particular places, like a dot on a map of the United States that represents "Chicago." It's much more complex.

"It's not like a simple map planted on her chest," says Kuiken. "It's fragmented. But it's very exciting that there's such fidelity. She can feel very fine touches. Touches as light as a pin on her chest. And she feels it as if it's in her hand."

Kuiken has found a way to express this new arrangement that helps most people understand it better. "Think about it [the skin on her chest] as hand skin," he says. "We took a nerve, the hand nerve, and just sent it to new skin."

It's taken time to discover the different places in that area on Claudia's chest that correspond to different parts of her hand. If you touch a certain place on the patch, she feels the pinky of her amputated hand—another place is her thumb. "It's as if her hand now lives in her chest," says Kuiken.

Kuiken compares the redirection of Claudia's nerves to the wiring of a telephone. "Let's say you call up your brother," he says. "You have a nice conversation. You hang up. He was in the living room. Okay, you call him back and now he's in the dining room on a different phone. You have a good conversation. You're talking to him. You don't know whether he's in the living room or the dining room—just like the brain doesn't know where that skin is."

Dr. Paul Marasco is a neuroscientist in Kuiken's group. He is recording all of the different sensations in Claudia's missing hand.

"She has distinct sensations of her joints being bent back in particular ways," says Marasco. "She has feelings of her skin being stretched."

Marasco's masterpiece is a map of all of Claudia's sensations and their corresponding locations on her chest. It's showing doctors how the brain deals with injury, and it's also helping to pave the way for future prosthetic technology. The new frontier? Sending messages from the artificial hand back to the brain.

A GRATEFUL CYBORG

Although tremendously excited by Claudia's case, Kuiken says it's hard to know how research will progress and exactly what he and his fellow pioneers in the field will be able to accomplish.

"Art and science intersect on the operating table," he explains. "You never know exactly what's going to happen. Often the game plan you've got in the beginning has to change. And that's okay. As long as you can creatively and intelligently decide how you're going to rewire people."

The success of Claudia's experience is pointing toward even more exciting developments. "We're doing an experiment where we have a sensor that can touch objects. And then a device that presses on her skin, proportional to that sensor. So if you tap something it'll tap on this skin and she'll feel like she's tapping her hand. And if you push it a little lighter, or rub it, that will be translated to the skin."

So it's possible to imagine the day when an artificial limb would be able to interpret sensations such as heat and cold?

"Absolutely," says Kuiken. "Someday we hope to have the sensors embedded in these new prostheses that can collect that information. So when you touch your hot cup of coffee, you know it's warm, and bring that information back to this reinnervated skin. Perhaps the most important part of the sensation feedback is psychological. When you touch something with this prosthetic hand, it will feel like your hand."

He spoke of an experiment in which the team came very close to what he'd described: "We were doing an experiment where we were sliding a prosthetic finger with the sensor across the table. We had a device that was pressing on the skin [of her chest]. Claudia could feel the direction in which that finger was sliding and the coarseness of the material underneath."

Claudia's brain had been thoroughly mapped before the surgery, and was again immediately afterward, and again for months after her recovery. "Now we're going back and re-mapping her brain to see how it's changed," says Kuiken. "And it's a very exciting glimpse into how the brain remodels itself—something we call plasticity."

Claudia is thrilled to be part of this discovery process and is dedicated to the research. She spends most of her vacations at Kuiken's laboratory, testing new equipment, like an advanced six-motor arm.

"For me, what's so exciting about the sensation on my chest is that we have the potential to get feedback, physical feedback, from a prosthesis. Because, right now, I can't tell you if my hand is grabbing anything unless I can see it. But we're testing constantly, trying to figure out how much vibration I can feel, how much pressure I can feel—what's the point at which I can discriminate?"

Claudia says that she was teased by her friends because she wasn't aware of *The Bionic Woman*, the television show from the 1970s starring Lindsay Wagner. Wagner played a woman who was given artificial limbs with superpowers. Claudia says she doesn't want special powers in her arm or hand, but she does think that there is no limit to what bionics in the future will be able to accomplish.

"A lot of what we do here sounds like science fiction," Kuiken says. "And what's exciting about it is that it's not going to be science *fiction* anymore. Fiction is going to drop off, and it's just science. Bionics have no limit. I don't think there are limits in what we can give back to people."

Kuiken's team is now working on getting this mind-controlled robotic arm to new military amputees. They've already performed the nerve transfer surgery on two soldiers at Walter Reed Army Medical Center. And they hope that these veterans will not only be able to use their new limbs, but, like Claudia, be able to feel their missing ones.

"I think sometimes I forget and I take for granted what I'm doing. And then all of a sudden, I realize, wow, there are people who haven't had the opportunity to be at this point yet. It just makes me take a deep breath and just thank God that I have been able to be part of this."

12. WHAT'S THAT SONG?

"**I WAS WORKING FULL-TIME, GOING TO SCHOOL FULL-TIME,**" SAYS Stacey Gayle. "Going to church, singing in the choir. Everything was great. I had big dreams."

Stacey took the subway every day to her job as a customer service representative in Manhattan—a normal, busy, productive life.

Her mother describes Stacey as a "good child" who didn't party too much—a mom's dream. Until that dream turned, for both mother and daughter, into something that began to resemble a nightmare.

In 2003, when she was twenty-one years old, Stacey began having epileptic seizures. Her doctors tried a battery of medications, but none of them worked. Each day, Stacey had as many as ten grand mal seizures, where she would collapse and convulse.

She'd feel the seizure coming on: "I'd get a certain aura, a certain smell. It's a weird smell—kind of like smelling salts—a strong perfume scent. And I'd get a certain feeling—I'd get nauseous."

The warning wasn't much help. "It happened so fast that I really didn't have time to do anything," Stacey says. "I'm already on the floor, knocked out."

The fear of having a seizure began to have a terrible impact on Stacey and her mother, Marhlan Nelson, who works in a Manhattan hotel.

Stacey was still living at home, and nights were particularly hard on her mother. "A lot of times I would not be able to sleep when I came home from work because I would just want her to stay in the room with me in the bed," she says. "So I would know exactly what was going on with her." And they never knew what was causing the seizures.

Gradually, her mother learned she didn't have to call an ambulance every time Stacey had a seizure. "I would just try to softly call her back," she says. "One of her doctors, Dr. Mehta, would say: speak softly to her, don't frighten her. Just turn her on her side, speak to her, keep calling her to get her to come around. And she would come around and [say] 'Mom, what happened?'"

The seizures changed Stacey's life. "Everything that I liked to do, I had to stop doing," she says. "I stopped going to school, stopped working, stopped going to church."

Her doctors were baffled by Stacey's seizures. And Stacey didn't have a clue as to what brought them on.

Then she went to a barbecue with friends. They were standing around, listening to music and talking, and the popular Sean Paul song "Temperature" began to play.

"I just remember falling and having a big seizure," Stacey recalls. She didn't think to connect the music to the seizure at that point. "I didn't think much of it, 'cause, you know, I was having seizures."

THE MUSIC CONNECTION

Stacey's doctors had told her that seizures are often triggered by a specific stimulus. If you find the trigger, you can better control the problem. Ms. Nelson, desperate to solve the mystery, was terrified that her daughter would have a seizure on a subway platform, for example, and fall into the path of an incoming train. She remembers telling Stacey: "This is a major problem, and we both have to start figuring out if it's my perfume, if it's your perfume . . ."

And then Stacey began to notice it. Whenever the Sean Paul song came on—the one she had heard at the barbecue—she had a seizure. It was too strange, though. Could it be the *song*? She felt there was a connection, and she told her mother—who was incredulous at first. But Stacey became increasingly certain that it was music—and not just "Temperature"—that was causing her seizures.

Mother and daughter were both deeply worried. "I love music a lot," says Ms. Nelson. "I was like—'Lord, have mercy.'"

Stacey was hesitant to tell her doctor her theory—that songs sent her into seizures. "I was hoping that he wouldn't check me into a mental institution," she says. "I definitely thought I was crazy."

ONE IN TEN MILLION

"I had heard of musicogenic epilepsy," says Dr. Ashesh Mehta, a neurosurgeon at Long Island Jewish Medical Center. "I'd certainly read about it, though I'd never seen a case myself.

Of course, given how rare it is, I was a little skeptical at first. The prevalence was something like one in ten million. I wanted to evaluate her."

Mehta said that Stacey's condition offered several keys that were helpful in the diagnosis. Stacey's self-described auras were a clue. "What Stacey was experiencing with her auras is just the very initial part of the seizure," says Mehta. "The fact that she has them tells us that it's probably partial epilepsy, coming from one little area of the brain. It's not the whole brain going off at once. If that were the case, she'd have no warning." The *type* of aura was also informative. "The type of auras that she had—smells, tastes—are often related to temporal lobe seizures," he adds. "More clues that these seizures were coming from one little area of the brain."

Mehta narrowed the search to a structure in the right side of the brain, the hippocampus. "Focal epilepsy is often [in] the hippocampus," he says. "The hippocampus is often the culprit."

Located in the temporal lobe, the hippocampus is—ta dahh!—where music is processed. It is also involved with memory. Mehta explains: "There is a closeness of the two structures that normally process music and this area that's important for memory."

Mehta thinks the areas that process music send signals to the area that remembers the music and is also involved with emotional responses to music. This process went awry in Stacey's case. "Somehow, a connection formed between a particular pattern of activity that represented music in her brain and another pattern of activity which represented seizures," he says. "One of the things we know about the brain is that there's something called association. When two patterns of brain activity occur at the same time, the next time one happens, the likelihood of the other one happening is increased."

Mehta absolves Sean Paul of any fault—he didn't cause Stacey's initial epileptic seizure. She had developed epilepsy, and she also listened to a lot of music. Somehow, in Stacey's brain, the pattern of activity that represented music became associated with another pattern of activity that caused her seizures.

"The two patterns of activity were coincident," says Mehta.

At some point, when that very popular Sean Paul song was being played, Stacey happened to have a seizure, and somehow, an association occurred in her brain.

"So that the next time that pattern of activity occurred, the seizures were also likely to occur," says Mehta. "That's my theory, but there's really no way to prove this thing," he admits. "It's still a mystery."

TESTING, TESTING

But Mehta needed more proof before he could design a strategy for treatment.

First, Mehta ordered an electroencephalogram, or EEG, to record the brain's signals. Electrical leads were placed on Stacey's scalp in the hospital. Three or four days of EEG testing passed, but Stacey did not have a seizure. She had plans to visit her aunt in Jamaica and had a plane to catch. She was going to be in the hospital for one more day, and she said, "Well, why don't I bring in my iPod? I can make myself have the seizure."

It seemed a little odd, but Mehta agreed. And the results were immediate—in the hospital bed, with the electrodes stuck all over her head, Stacey turned her iPod on. She had three seizures in one night.

Delighted to be closer to an answer, she insisted on making her flight to Jamaica the following day. Unfortunately, when she got to the terminal at JFK, the airport bar was playing music. She had a seizure and missed her flight.

"I think that that was a real wake-up call for her," Mehta says.

Stacey agrees: "I just had to get these seizures under control."

Next stop: the hospital's PET (positron-emission tomography) scan suite.

"We brought her iPod in, and we hooked up the EEG leads, and we played the music," says Mehta. And Stacey immediately had a seizure, caught by both an EEG recording and the PET scan. It was a breakthrough: this test narrowed down the area of origin for the seizures.

"It actually showed a little area of the brain where the seizures might be coming from," says Mehta. They were "fairly convinced" the seizures were originating in the temporal lobe, an area of the neocortex. But what part of that temporal lobe, and were there other lobes in the brain involved as well?

To determine this, Mehta implanted, directly into Stacey's brain, electrodes attached to an EEG. It was the only way to determine precisely where the seizures originated.

"Again, we had the same problem," says Mehta. "We couldn't get any seizures. Until we put the iPod on. Then she had, again, three seizures when we started the music. And they all came from one area of the brain."

WHAT IS EPILEPSY?

A digression for a moment about epilepsy—a medical condition that typically involves recurrent seizures. "A lot of people will have seizures at some point [in their lives]," Mehta says. "But they won't come back again. In fact, one in ten people will have a seizure at some point. Epilepsy represents a condition where patients have seizures over and over again. They don't go away. And that affects maybe one percent of the population." Let me translate that: about three million Americans.

Mehta explains that the seizures result from an abnormal pattern of electrical activity in the brain. It may start in the whole brain at once, or in only one part, spreading to the rest of the brain over the course of minutes. Seizure are sometimes accompanied by convulsions and sometimes characterized by something as subtle as staring into space.

Mehta said that some people develop epilepsy in childhood, but it's not uncommon to develop epilepsy in young adulthood, in one's teens or twenties. Mehta has also had some patients who have developed epilepsy in their forties and fifties.

What causes it?

"It can be a result of many different conditions," says Mehta. "It could be a metabolic disturbance, it could be an abnormal lesion in the brain, an abnormal blood vessel, maybe even a tumor."

Mehta stresses the importance of figuring out the cause of a patient's seizures—the trigger. "Number one, to try to avoid it; number two, we try to design the therapy that would be most appropriate for it."

When Stacey first began having seizures, she could control them somewhat with medication. But Mehta explains that, before long, her seizures became "refractory." They could no longer be controlled with drugs.

SURGERY

Once Mehta had found the focal point of Stacey's seizures, he began to consider surgery. He says that he had to figure out whether he could take out the part of the brain that was causing the seizures without injuring or impairing Stacey. If the surgery was successful, could it help or, perhaps, even cure her seizures?

All surgery carries risk, and brain surgery carries unique types of risk. "We had to make sure," says Mehta, "that if we removed this small part of her brain on the right side, she would have memory on the other side of her brain."

How much of Stacey's brain would need to be removed to do the trick? Six centimeters of tissue. And tests showed Mehta he could remove this much of Stacey's brain without impacting her memory. Mehta was confident, "and we knew that we could do this safely," he says.

Convincing Stacey and her mother that removing a piece of Stacey's brain was a good idea? Another matter.

"They told me, okay, you have this trigger, I think you're a good candidate for surgery," says Stacey. "But when you hear 'brain surgery,' you think you're coming out paralyzed and a vegetable. So I was totally against it. I was like—'No, thank you. Is there any other way that we could go?'"

Mehta told Stacey surgery was the only option, and the chances of being free from seizures after surgery were 80 or 90 percent.

As things were, Stacey was not exactly enjoying much quality of life. Think about where you hear music—in malls, in grocery stores, in elevators, on television, in cabs, in friends' homes, in their cars . . . It's hard to escape it. And much of what Stacey loved in the world was musical.

"Music is really, really important in my life," she says. "I was getting really depressed," Stacey recalls, "and sometimes entertaining thoughts of suicide. Everything that I love was taken away from me."

Stacey thought long and hard about the operation and finally came to a decision. "I wanted to get my life back on track, so I decided that I really needed to do it," she says.

The day of the surgery Stacey was frightened. "I was extremely nervous," she says. "Words can't describe how I felt. But I had a lot of trust in my doctors."

The oddest thing about her surgery: as in many operations on the brain, Stacey was conscious throughout the procedure. Brain surgeons need to occasionally ask the patient to speak or identify pictures to make sure that they're not damaging vital areas. She came through it perfectly—and as often happens after brain surgery, remembers nothing of the procedure.

"I just remember Dr. Mehta was telling me afterwards that I was laughing during surgery. That was good to know."

AFTERMATH

Stacey went home three days after the operation. It was time to test whether or not the surgery had worked. Stacey and her mom were nervous, almost giddy. "She started laughing, and I was laughing," says Ms. Nelson.

"I want to try it," Stacey told her mom. "I want to see what it is. I want to feel it."

Stacey found "Temperature" on her iPod. "I was nervous at first," she recalls. "I was extremely nervous, actually. When I first turned on the music, my heart was racing so fast, knowing that every time I had listened to that song before I would have a seizure."

But she played the music and . . . sat, delighted, normal, in her chair!

"For the first time in five years!" she says.

She called Mehta immediately to let him know the good news.

Mehta thinks more epileptics could be helped by surgery.

"If we just do the numbers, in terms of the prevalence of epilepsy in the population, and the prevalence of intractable epilepsy like Stacey had, I would estimate maybe about a hundred fifty thousand people, just in the United States, would benefit from it," Mehta says.

Stacey and her mother couldn't be happier that she decided to take that chance. Her mother, who lived with Stacey's condition for five years, is enormously relieved.

"I cannot explain what life is like today," says Ms. Nelson. "I can go to work, and I don't feel nervous, like I'm gonna get a call from the hospital that she's having a seizure and you need to come get your daughter."

Stacey and her mother are taking each day as it comes.

"And we're thanking God," says Ms. Nelson. "Stacey is very happy. I can tell because she has been doing a lot of shopping! She goes by herself, with her friends, and she goes to school by herself. She calls me when she's in school just to let me know that she's okay. She's just happy. I can tell."

"I feel good!" says Stacey. "I go in the store and smile, and they must be thinking I'm crazy. I'm like, 'Yeah, I'm in here!'" Muzak blaring.

And once again, her iPod is her friend. "I always have my iPod with me, twenty-four seven!" she says. "I always have the radio on. In the shower, I have the radio on. It feels amazing just to be able to listen to music. As soon as I get in my car, I turn on the music. I come home, I put on the music. BET, MTV—all those channels. I'm back! Back to church. Back in the choir. Back to school. Life is good. No complaints!"

What does she have to say about "Temperature" these days?

"That's one hot song."

13. PIZZA PARALYSIS

A MEDICAL CASE IS A GIANT JIGSAW PUZZLE—SYMPTOMS, GENETICS, medicines, side effects. Which symptoms mean something? Which can you ignore? How much does the family history have to do with the case? The list is endless. We loved La Ron Young's case because it showed us that every tiny component is important when a medical mystery shows up.

When La Ron was a student at Cal State Northridge, he woke up on the first day of school in his sophomore year to find that he could barely move. His arms and legs seemed not to function—he was overcome with a debilitating weakness. It was so strange that his girlfriend at the time thought he was putting her on.

"I'm a playful person, and she thought I was playing," says La Ron. "She was like, 'Stop playing.' I was like, 'No one is playing. I'm being for real. I can't move!'"

La Ron, an active African-American student who had been able to play a game of basketball the night before, was almost completely paralyzed. The same guy who had gone out for beer and pizza after the game could now only roll out of bed and crash to the floor, smashing onto his face, lying helpless.

There was no talk of playing after that.

One frantic 911 call later, he was rushed to Lancaster Community Hospital's ER by ambulance. He told the ER staff that he was paralyzed and feeling sick.

Then his heart stopped. "I went flatline. I was feeling real sleepy, and I hear a voice say, 'La Ron, can you hear me?' They were like, 'Cough for me. If you want to stay alive, cough!'"

La Ron was able to cough "real soft."

"Keep coughing," he remembers the doctors saying. "They were like your coach at the finish line, telling you: 'Don't give up, you can keep going; come on, cough for me!'"

The doctors were able to restart La Ron's heart, and his paralysis eventually decreased. After a battery of tests, the doctors were only sure of one thing: his blood work showed that La Ron had dangerously low potassium levels. They infused him with potassium and, mystified, kept this otherwise healthy young man in the hospital for three weeks for observation, then sent him home. With no diagnosis, he just continued with his life, coasting along with no explanation of what had happened to him. He had episodes of minor muscle weakness, but nothing like the paralysis that sent him crashing to the floor and caused his heart to stop. He went on about his life.

And then it came back.

A MAN TRAPPED IN HIS OWN BODY

La Ron says he and his pals threw a "game night. Taboo, Jester, you know, a bunch of games, a bunch of friends, having fun. We ordered pizza, banana cream pie, ice cream. Being college students, we eat a lot of junk food. About maybe one or two o'clock I feel weak. I went to bed, woke up the next morning, my muscles real weak. It feels like you go to the gym and work out so much, the next day you feel like putty. Like your muscles are shot. There's no energy."

He was "out of it," paralyzed, and one of La Ron's roommates ran him over to UCLA's Medical Center, where he was first examined by the ER staff and then seen by Dr. Peter Balingit, an internist.

La Ron's case was a true medical mystery to his doctors: why would an otherwise healthy young man experience sudden paralysis? There was no trauma, no neck injury. When the doctor examined him, La Ron was able to blink on command, move his neck, and breathe normally, but he couldn't move his arms or legs. He was unable to get up off the examination table by himself or walk, but aside from La Ron's muscular weakness, he seemed in reasonably good shape. Balingit says he was alert, oriented, and able to respond to questions.

"He seemed very calm but definitely anxious because he was almost like a man trapped in his own body," Balingit recalls.

Balingit learned that during the last several months, La Ron had been to both Mexico and Africa. The doctor thought that, because La Ron was young, in generally good health, and had been traveling, he might have been exposed to some sort of toxin. Or had he been bitten by a tick that carries a poison that causes nerve paralysis?

"Additionally," says Balingit, "with his weakness we were also entertaining the diagnosis of Guillain-Barré syndrome, an autoimmune phenomenon where basically your body attacks the nervous system, and that causes paralysis and can lead to respiratory failure."

Balingit also had to consider multiple sclerosis, where the protective sheaths around the nerves wear away. It has some of the same symptoms: weakness, unusual sensations, and visual complaints. Or was it a seizure disorder, which can cause muscle rigidity, even when the patient is alert and aware of his surroundings? Balingit considered alcohol, drug use, and certain medications, particularly colchicine, which is used for gout and may cause symmetric weakness. And that wasn't even counting the more exotic possible causes for La Ron's condition—like the ingestion of toxins from a puffer fish in improperly prepared sashimi. Balingit also wanted to make sure La Ron didn't have a spinal cord tumor or transverse myelitis—a cut or hemorrhage in the spinal cord that can come from a routine sports injury. How to tease out the real culprit? Symptoms, tests, and the patient's own history. In short: ask every question you can think of.

Balingit began to rule out the various possibilities. Guillain-Barré usually begins with an upper respiratory infection and tends to start in the legs and ascend upward. La Ron's symptoms didn't fit that pattern. A careful exam didn't reveal the presence of any ticks on La Ron's scalp or body, and he hadn't been hiking or camping in the local mountains, so that probably wasn't the cause. La Ron wasn't a candidate for a spinal tumor, he didn't report any cancer warning signs (weight loss, for instance). As far as a hemorrhage or cut in the spinal cord, he told Balingit that he hadn't been in any accidents recently, lifted anything heavy, or experienced a fall—all common ways that hemorrhage can happen.

Sometimes spinal cord injuries may be caused by infections, but, typically, says Balingit, "those patients have a history of IV drug use or have some sort of portal of infection for bacteria to enter. This patient was definitely an upstanding young man and denied any type of illicit drug use . . . He hadn't eaten any new foods, wasn't really a big fan of sushi, and denied being started on medications for gout. Sometimes cholesterol-lowering medications can cause weakness, but again, given that he was very young, he hadn't been exposed to these medications. We quickly decided that these possibilities were less likely in this man."

THE QUESTION THEY DIDN'T ASK

The ER doctors drew an electrolyte panel, paying particular attention to La Ron's potassium, calcium, and sodium levels. They found, just as in La Ron's last debilitating episode, that he had very low potassium, so low it was almost life-threatening. That's extremely unusual in someone with a regular diet who isn't on a medication that affects potassium. Balingit also found that La Ron's thyroid was working overtime: he had too much thyroid hormone in his blood.

"Once we discovered that his potassium level was low," says Balingit, "we ordered oral doses of potassium, which failed to improve his symptoms. So our treating team was more aggressive and gave intravenous administrations of potassium over two days. Once the potassium level corrected, his muscle weakness improved. He was able to move, walk, sit up. With respect to his overactive thyroid, we decided to give a trial of medications called beta-blockers, which are normally used for heart disease or hypertension."

This combination of treatments allowed La Ron to recover and return to a state of good health. But doctors still didn't know why his potassium levels had plummeted or his thyroid was overactive. Balingit and his team sifted through the medical literature for any syndrome with muscle weakness, paralysis, low potassium, high thyroid. They came up with a group of conditions called periodic paralysis. But the one that fit La Ron's case best was most common in those people with Asian ancestry.

That led to a true "lightbulb moment." It came because they asked a couple of simple questions: what had you been eating, and who are your parents?

Balingit explains: "After taking a more careful history, we were able to find out that just prior to admission [to the ER] he had consumed a large amount of pizza, in essence a very large carbohydrate load. That and the fact [of] the patient's ethnic background—certain diseases do tend to run with certain ethnicities—a hyperactive thyroid and low potassium, all these things tied together really clinched the diagnosis of what we call hyperthyroid periodic paralysis [HPP]."

La Ron looks African-American, so his ethnicity seemed obvious. But nobody had *asked* him about his ethnic group. La Ron's father is Filipino—which turned out to be the key: the question they hadn't asked. His Asian ancestry clinched it.

"I think sometimes we physicians don't utilize basic history-taking, physical exam skills as we did just years ago, and now rely on more high-tech, heavy-duty tests," Balingit comments. "In this case, perhaps if we were more vigilant in asking about his habits and his background, we might have been able to make this diagnosis sooner."

La Ron was suffering from what, in layman's terms, could be called pizza paralysis. HPP comes two basic ways: hypokalemic, low-potassium periodic paralysis and hyperkalemic, high-potassium periodic paralysis. Both cause ions to move around your cells in unusual ways. When that happens, you get muscle weakness or uncoordinated muscle contraction. Here are the triggers: eating a high carbohydrate load, cold weather, excessive exercise, and alcohol or drug use. Pizza, beer, basketball . . .

"Typically you would treat this type of periodic paralysis by recommending that the patient avoid cold weather, avoid excess alcohol intake, avoid large carbohydrate loads to help prevent further occurrences of these episodes of weakness," says Balingit.

When you have HPP, your potassium levels cause the muscle problems.

Balingit: "If potassium does not move in or out of the cell in a synchronized fashion, that leads to disorganized contraction. In our patient's case, he admitted having a large carbohydrate load, mainly a large pizza, before retiring for the evening. It is well documented that when a patient takes in a large carbohydrate load, that stimulates insulin production. Insulin helps drive a lot of carbohydrates, in the form of sugars, into muscles and body tissue. What [it] also takes in with [it] is potassium. Patients with periodic paralysis have difficulty processing this potassium load. That can cause unorganized contraction and lead to weakness. So that was our hypothesis as far as why this patient ate a large carbohydrate load and then very shortly [afterward] developed paralysis."

PART OF LIFE

Once the diagnosis was made, facts fell into place. La Ron realized that some of his relatives on his father's side had the same condition—in a less crippling form.

"My grandma and my auntie, they take K-Lor because of low potassium," says La Ron (although they don't experience the sudden drops in potassium levels that he does).

La Ron now takes a pill to stabilize his potassium levels. "It's huge," he says of the pill's size. "It looks like a horse pill."

La Ron has his condition pretty much under control, though it has affected his life. Not just because he can longer eat massive amounts of pizza, or because he tries to eat lots of potassium-rich foods like bananas and potatoes. "I go to the doctors, they tell me, 'Just be normal, try to do normal things,'" he says. "But it's kind of difficult, because I used to break-dance, and I'm scared to. It's very harsh on your body, especially depending on what kind of break-dancer you are. What type of moves you do. Floor moves do with your muscles. Sweating, you lose a lot of potassium. So I slowed down and stopped break-dancing. I don't do shows anymore. So [my condition] has killed my love for dancing."

Perhaps even more distressing for a player like La Ron—his condition has impacted his love life. "It's kind of hard to explain to a young lady [that] I have a disease," he says. "I have to go through a whole story. And they don't really understand. They're like, 'Are you serious? I've never heard of that before.' I have to explain that it's a rare disease usually found in people of Asian descent. And they kind of look at me, like, well, you're African-American. I am African-American, but my dad is Filipino.

"It's like you're dealing with diabetes or high blood pressure," La Ron says. "You have a routine. You take your pills in the morning, you take your pills in the afternoon. If you feel it's coming on, you might want to boost your potassium by eating a few more bananas or drinking orange juice. It's part of life now."

The take-home for all of us? When your doctors take your "history," tell them *everything you can think of.* You don't know what tiny fact is going to be the key: your mom's migraines, your love of orange juice . . . We were astonished to find that a diagnosis can hang on a Filipino father and a pizza.

14. LOCKED IN

Some of the syndromes we research let us explore the amazing ways the brain works, or the complicated, miraculous way fetuses develop in the womb. With "locked-in syndrome," though, we ended up not only amazed at what can happen in the human *body*, but in awe of the resiliency of the human spirit and the capacity of the human heart.

Imagine lying inert, unmoving, totally paralyzed. Your only way of telling people "I'm not dead!" is the tiny blink of one eye. You are trapped in your body, and nobody knows you're "there." We interviewed two people who've lived it.

GLENDA AND KEVIN HICKEY

Glenda Hickey of Leduc, Alberta, in Canada, was in the kitchen with a blinding headache. She picked up the phone to call her husband, Kevin, at work, and fell to the floor—a stroke had stopped blood flowing to her brain. Glenda had hit her nose on the way down and was bleeding. Her daughter, Kaitlin, not quite three at the time, knew that something was wrong with Mommy and wanted to help.

"I found all these Band-Aids, and I tried putting them all over her face so the bleeding would stop," says Kaitlin, who was nine when we interviewed her.

In the meantime, Kevin was trying to call home, but Glenda's call had taken the phone off the hook. At first, her husband was aggravated. Then worried. He called a neighbor to check on his wife. The neighbor discovered Glenda motionless on the kitchen floor, Kaitlin beside her.

Kevin recalls the nightmarish scenario when he raced to the hospital. "They were doing tests on her. They were rubbing their knuckles on her chest quite hard to see if she'd respond. And she just would look straight ahead. She just couldn't respond."

Doctors suspected that Glenda might already be brain-dead. But she was fully aware, locked into a body that had become a prison. With every mental faculty intact—she could see, hear, reason, feel—she was completely paralyzed. None of her doctors yet suspected it, but Glenda had become one of only a few hundred patients worldwide to have "locked-in syndrome."

Dr. Stanley Tuhrim, professor of neurology and director of the Mount Sinai Stroke Center in New York, says that the locked-in state is "incredibly terrifying and incredibly frustrating. Unable to move. Unable to communicate. Locked in with one's own thoughts. Most patients in this condition don't survive or don't recover enough to tell us what their inner thoughts are."

The particular sort of stroke that causes the syndrome is different from other strokes in two ways: location and severity. A blood clot works its destructive way deep into the basilar artery, in the brain stem near the base of the neck, the area of the brain that functions as a kind of relay station between our thoughts and our movements. The brain, still conscious and alert, can keep issuing commands, but the body can no longer follow them.

"For some reason, a lot of the total occlusions of the basilar artery seem to occur in relatively young people," says Tuhrim. "There are a variety of causes for the type of stroke that causes the syndrome. One of the more common is an embolus, a blood clot that forms in the heart and then breaks off and travels up to the basilar artery, lodging there and preventing blood flow beyond that area. Sometimes there's atherosclerosis, which gradually narrows the basilar artery. Then, perhaps, an embolus forms in the heart or elsewhere and travels up and lodges in the area that's already narrowed by the atherosclerotic changes."

KEVIN JUST HAD A FEELING that his wife was fully conscious, although she couldn't move or respond. He says he somehow knew Glenda was "there," and he discovered that she could blink her eyes in response to his questions. Doctors were astonished to find the sort of case you only read about in textbooks. Eventually, Glenda learned to communicate by moving her eyes up for yes and down for no, and using a letter board to spell out words and phrases. Kevin would call out "a, b, c, d," and when he hit the right letter, she would signal yes with her eyes. Now it's streamlined: that alphabetical chart has grouped the letters into rows—first she signals a row number, then the letter. By now the whole family has memorized the chart.

Glenda is back at home with her family and an aide who looks after her for fourteen hours a day while Kevin works.

The Hickeys' marriage is strong—though you'd think they might wilt under these circumstances. Glenda may be "locked in," but she's not left out. "Glenda and I both work together, and we both understand what has to happen each day as a team, as husband and wife, as Batman and Robin, whoever," says Kevin. "We made the decision together to get through this. If one of us feels that we're not pulling our weight, just falling asleep at the wheel, then it's not going to work, because everybody has to be on board. We both kick each other in the butt every now and then for being a little lackadaisical or whatever. If one person runs it too much, that person just fails."

STEVE AND CINDY CHIAPPA

It was the same for Steve Chiappa of Toms River, New Jersey—a hard-driving businessman who ran a multimillion-dollar company that managed parking lots.

He overheard the doctors tell his wife Cindy that he was a vegetable—and he couldn't even whisper, "I'm still here."

Steve and Cindy, high school sweethearts, were on their way to a Christmas Eve dinner. Steve said he wasn't feeling well, then collapsed. He'd had a stroke in the car—a stroke that would have the same incredibly rare outcome as Glenda's. When he woke in the hospital, he even heard the staff telling Cindy that the blinking of his eyes—his increasingly desperate attempt to communicate—was just a reflex. She says that doctors told her, "He's not going to ever eat, ever walk . . . Maybe he'll open his eyes. He is not going to be more than a vegetable."

Steve heard a doctor suggest to Cindy that they disconnect his pacemaker, which had been implanted years before.
Cindy recalls the doctor saying: "If something happens, it
happens. That might be an easy way for him to go."

She also recalls her immediate response. "I was pissed,"
says Cindy. "I was really angry. I said, 'I don't want you anywhere near him. I want you off this case. Get out of my
sight.'"

Steve recalls the incident in a book he is now writing.
Here's an excerpt, as he recalls the doctor's words and his
own desperate thoughts:

> "He can't understand. I know you want to believe it, but
> it just isn't so. It really isn't a bad way to go."
>
> Had I remembered our last anniversary? Had I been
> a good husband? Had I told her how much I loved her? I
> guess so. She was yelling, "You stay away from him, I
> don't want you near my husband. He can understand. . . .
> My husband is coming home with me."

Cindy "decoded" Steve's blinks and realized he was completely aware. After five years and tremendous physical effort, Steve has worked his way back from the stroke that
locked him in. With intensive therapy and hard work on his
part, he is now able to use a remote to control a television
and computer. Is he a vegetable? "Sure," he jokes, "a thinking
vegetable." He is outfitted with a special wheelchair and
mobile. He has even learned to speak again. And he's the first
to say that for a while after his stroke, he wanted to die. He was
consumed by anger and self-pity. Why me? he asked. What
did I do wrong?

"Kill me," he blinked out to Cindy more than once. "You have to help me. I can't do it myself."

Then he began to look around him—at the wife and family that still loved him, even though his body and the personality inside no longer "matched." Steve says that was what really saved him—they made him understand that he truly *was* still "himself."

Two reflexes are his most precious: his ability to laugh and to cry. He tells Cindy: "It takes just as much energy to laugh as to cry, so you might as well laugh."

Steve says that every night in his dreams, he gets up, walks, goes to work. "I can dream it," he says. He acknowledges that it's tough to stay positive, particularly facing financial ruin. "We went through all our savings," says Cindy. "All our businesses, our houses, everything. It's all gone."

"I fight getting down every day," Steve says. "But I get through it."

Our television crew watched, deeply moved, as he asked his wife for a kiss and then more kisses, and she happily obliged, showering him with love and affection. Yes, Steve's case was a medical mystery, but it was also a love story.

LOVE AND "LOCKED-IN"

As is Kevin and Glenda's. The commitment Kevin and Glenda made to each other as husband and wife still extends to the bedroom. Yes, she can only communicate letter by letter, but Kevin says he does his best to please his wife, who, although paralyzed, *feels* everything. "You try being in total control with your wife where she is just lapping up the love," he says. "You do everything for her for fifteen minutes and the sweat pours off you. That's a major workout. You won't have to go to the gym for a week."

If you're shocked that their relationship still remains intimate, Kevin has an immediate comeback. He's puzzled that people would assume the couple's love life would change simply because of Glenda's condition. "We [both] understand that we love each other. I know my wife's totally mentally cognitive. She always said no before, so she still says no."

When he makes this joke, Glenda, who, after years of therapy is able to make sounds, laughs.

Perhaps the most extraordinary part of this couple's story is the fact that their enduring intimacy has led to the birth of their third child, a daughter named Hope.

That's right, in her locked-in state, Glenda became pregnant and carried a baby full-term.

"One of those hot August summer nights," says Kevin. "It was her fault."

How so?

"Sometime you'll have to try this with your husband," he replies. "Make him spell something that he normally wouldn't spell and see what his reaction is to it. Spell 'please touch me here.' Don't say it—spell it slowly. [It gives] a new meaning to intimacy."

Spelling as an aphrodisiac? "Yeah, it's fun," Kevin admits. "Sometimes I get halfway through spelling, and I have to stop because you're sick of spelling. 'Okay, I know what you want!' "

Glenda says she could tell she was pregnant. The doctors tried to dissuade the couple from having a sister for Kaitlin. But their can-do approach overcame whatever reservations they had. Glenda, because of her history of stroke, had to have blood thinner shots twice a day. The process was expensive, straining the couple's already stretched budget.

"By the time we finished," says Steve, "it was about thirty thousand dollars in extra costs."

According to the doctors, the labor and delivery by C-section were routine. The doctor delivering Hope had been a naysayer about the prospect of Glenda being able to bring another child into the world. But Kevin remembers him saying after the delivery: "You know, I think God had a little hand in this one."

Kevin has had a crash course in hands-on mothering. "I didn't realize the work that you have to do," he says. "Not having any sleep. Awake every four hours. Being Mom is only for moms. Not for dads."

"You had never done that before?" we asked Kevin.

"No."

At this point, Glenda spells out the word: "Exciting."

"I felt pretty comfortable," says Kevin. "I knew Glenda could help me and tell me what was right and what was wrong like she always does. And we'd get through it."

Their baby's name resonates on many levels for the Hickeys, not the least of which is the hope that Glenda will one day recover.

"What day is it going to happen?" says Kevin. "I married a woman with a million-dollar smile, everything that I wanted in a wife or a friend."

Glenda guffaws. Kevin pays her no mind.

"She's been stripped of some of the things that she had before," he continues. "But she's gained others. I still wait for that one morning when the sun comes up and we resume."

That does not mean that the Hickeys are counting on it. Quite the contrary. They are, to an extraordinary degree, living in the moment.

"We're on earth to enjoy the things that are here," says Kevin. "To appreciate life as it is today."

NEITHER OF THESE COUPLES got the life they'd planned—but they seem to find joy in the life they're living. And they say, in the end, that is all anyone can ask for.

15. SURFER'S SYNDROME

Who would ever think that a young, healthy person riding a surfboard for the first time could be seriously hurt? Not in the way you'd think—a pulled muscle, a torn rotator cuff. This medical mystery is far more life-changing. One minute, you're riding the waves. Hours later, you're riding in a wheelchair, wondering if you'll ever walk again.

That was what happened to Joe Guintu, a twenty-four-year-old athlete who had played basketball in college and was always ready for a pickup game. He was in Hawaii with his girlfriend, Ivette Flores, for a family wedding in March 2007. Like many tourists, the couple decided to go surfing.

While Ivette had done a little surfing before, Joe hadn't, and he needed a lesson. They found an instructor, rented boards, and took a couple of minutes working things out on the sand—Joe, Ivette, and a couple of others who were also taking lessons. Then they headed for the water.

Joe proved to be a natural. "On my first try," he says, "I jump up on the board, and I'm like, whoa, this is fun! I get to the end of the wave. I jumped off the board [and] noticed something wasn't right."

Joe thought the discomfort he was beginning to feel came from asking his body to do something it hadn't done before. His back was sore, but he didn't take it seriously. "I assumed that it's my first time surfing, and I'm doing some strenuous activities, the twisting, the jumping . . . I paddle again. I get up, I surf it out and jump off, and again I noticed that strange feeling in my back. It wasn't pain, it was just sort of discomfort. It didn't hurt. But it didn't feel right."

He and Ivette decided to call it a day and went out to lunch. Joe assumed the feeling would pass. Instead, his legs were beginning to spasm. The couple decided to Jacuzzi at a hotel down the block.

"I did not want to walk to that hotel," Joe says. "I was in too much pain. But I sucked it up, and we walked over. And that was probably the last long walk that I took."

WHEN JOE'S CONDITION did not improve, Ivette insisted they find a doctor. As they waited to see someone at the clinic, Joe didn't think anything serious was going on: "I was thinking—it will be a day or two or three maybe. They'll give me some medicine and take the pain away and it will be fine."

A doctor listened to Joe's story and called in Dr. Beau Nakamoto, a neurologist. It was lucky that Nakamoto was the doctor who saw Joe. He's one of the few doctors familiar with this rare syndrome. After he ran a few neurological tests, he told Joe they were going to transport him to the hospital.

Joe was shocked: "I was thinking to myself, 'Are you serious? I went surfing and now my back hurts. What's going on?'"

A surfer has a greater chance of being attacked by a shark than being stricken with what Nakamoto calls "surfer's myelopathy." And there was no time to waste. In the worst case, Nakamoto knew, Joe could become paraplegic. He rushed Joe by ambulance to Straub Hospital in Honolulu.

JOE'S PARENTS were about to board a plane back to Los Angeles when they got the call that Joe was in the hospital. They arrived at Straub to find their son was about to get an MRI.

"While I was in the emergency room before the MRI," says Joe, "they kept on asking me to move my legs [and] toes." Joe easily completed both these tasks; he was still unconvinced that anything was seriously wrong. By this time, Nakamoto had told him the worst-case scenario: paralysis.

"Who encounters the worst-case scenario?" Joe remembers thinking. "Maybe there will be some residual pain. I'll take pills; everything will be fine. Whatever."

The MRI did not, however, paint a rosy picture. It showed that Joe's spinal cord was swollen and inflamed from the T-6 vertebra all the way through to his tailbone. And the situation was deteriorating rapidly.

"I distinctly remember after the MRI, when I got back to that emergency room, they asked me to move my toes, move my leg and all that," Joe says. "And that was the first time I couldn't . . . I couldn't do it."

"This story is stereotypical," says Nakamoto. "Visitor to Hawaii goes surfing for the first time, develops low back pain, comes out of the water, feels that their legs are weak, can't urinate. And then, over the next hour or so, has varying degrees of weakness. The story is always the same. It's a very rare condition. It affects only first-time surfers. We don't have a lot of information about this disorder. We never get follow-up because these people are all visitors to Hawaii. I see usually about two, maybe three cases per year, and that doesn't include my colleagues or the other neurologists in the community."

Dr. James Pearce, the neurologist who identified the first few cases of surfer's myelopathy in Hawaii, is a colleague of Nakamoto's. He describes the injury as "a mechanical problem. First-time surfers tend to lay flat on their board. They're excited about catching some waves. So they're always arching their backs to look up and see where the waves are coming from."

Pearce says this causes repeated hyperextension of their back, either through arching the back up straight or perhaps arching it up to one side or the other. For a very small percentage of first-time surfers, that hyperextension of the back—repeated again and again—causes an interruption in the blood supply to the spine.

Why does it happen to some first-time surfers and not others?

"We really don't know," said Pearce. "Some people think that it has to do with congestion in the veins around the spinal cord. Other people think that it has to do with kinking of one of the arteries that goes to the spinal cord."

IVETTE WAS WITH JOE in the ER after he learned the results of the MRI. She remembers feeling as though what was happening wasn't quite real. "It's a very surreal thing. Nothing happened. You went surfing. You just went *surfing*. And then to hear an hour later [that] you may never walk again . . . It's unbelievable."

Nakamoto tried to go easy on Joe. "When he told me about the MRI," Joe remembers, "I was asking him about the rest of my Hawaii trip. He said: 'Maybe we'll keep you for a night or two and then you can probably go to your hotel and head [home].' Later on he told me: 'Joe, right now you can't move your legs and it's not gonna be a day, a week, a month. It's gonna be at least a few months—*if ever*—that you'll walk again.'"

Joe's response was an indication of how he would meet the challenge over time. "I took it in stride. It didn't scare me. I looked at him with my poker face and said, 'All right.'"

MIKE FRITSCHNER

Mike Fritschner went to the same high school as Joe, though they never met. They have something else in common. It was the summer of 2006 and Mike and his family were on a cruise. Mike, fifteen years old, at six-four and 210 pounds, was a natural athlete, a high school sophomore who had already made varsity football.

While in the islands, Mike and his father decided to take surfing lessons. They spent about ten minutes with the instructor on the sand before taking their rented boards into the water.

"I was probably out there for twenty minutes," says Mike. "I stood up on one leg. I felt a little pop in my back. It was almost like a morning stretch thing. You stretch a little, and you hear everything crack. I wasn't really worried about it."

Mike tried to catch another wave. "I was paddling back out, and then I tried to get up again. This time it really started to hurt. It felt terrible, like somebody was crunching my backbone. I told my dad and the instructor that I was going in because my back really hurt. Even then I wasn't really worried about it."

Mike lay down on the sand and tried to stretch out his back. "I was doing some legs-to-chest stretches; I curled up in a ball. It just started to hurt ridiculously. My legs—there was something wrong with them. They felt tired, like I'd just run a mile."

Mike could barely walk by the time his father, Walt, helped him up off the beach. Then Mike's legs gave way completely.

"I totally collapsed," says Mike. "I could still feel my legs, but they were way too tired to move."

PROGNOSIS

According to Pearce, the prognosis for surfer's myelopathy varies. "I think we can sort the prognosis into two rough categories," he says. "We see some people that develop mild weakness. They stay ambulatory but still come to the emergency room."

Cases of mild weakness often do very well and completely recover; others aren't so lucky.

For people such as Joe and Mike, the prognosis is much grimmer. "If the person is totally paraplegic by the time they get to the emergency room, it's rare that they recover function," says Pearce. "We've had one or two cases in which profound weakness persisted for a number of weeks, and then they regained some of their strength."

It seems there is no middle ground for people who sustain this particular injury. "It's either a mild, benign syndrome or a really tragic case," says Pearce.

In general, if the individual is still working hard in physical therapy a year or two after the accident, and they are still not walking, the chances of anything like a full recovery are very slim.

Pearce says he sees three or four new cases a year. He says that the faster the patient gets out of the water and gets help, the better the prognosis, the greater the chances of walking again. But there is no surgery to correct the damage, no medication to turn things around.

While neurologists in Hawaiian hospitals recognize the injury, even among surfing instructors and lifeguards (people who ought to be on the lookout for it), it's pretty much unknown. The surfers and surfing instructors we talked to on the beach had never heard of "surfer's syndrome."

COURAGEOUS YOUNG MEN

Joe and Ivette, who married and live in Culver City, Colorado, have been working hard to remedy the lack of awareness about surfer's myelopathy in the surfing community.

They have started a foundation to offer support and information to others who, like Joe, take their first surfing lesson and walk out of the water into a wheelchair.

"We've made it a mission," says Ivette. "Friends of mine have helped me get this program off the ground."

Joe and Ivette have big plans for the Surfer's Myelopathy Foundation. "We want to educate people," says Ivette, "and help future, potential surfer's myelopathy patients decrease their likelihood of having such a severe prognosis."

Ivette describes the kind of advice and information they plan to make available. "If you get out of the water sooner rather than later, you might be better the next day," she says. "You might lose some sensation, but it might come back in a couple days, instead of having to go through a grueling recovery process. We want to teach the surfing instructors about this. No one knows about it. You talk to surfers, avid surfers, they've never heard of it. They're shocked. We want to go into the surfing schools in Hawaii and then hopefully later on in California and other places that are known for having a lot of first-time surfing lessons and teach instructors about risk factors and about what to do if they think someone may have it."

Ivette also says she wants instructors to issue warnings that there are other ways to be injured surfing aside from a shark attack or being hit by a board in the surf.

With physical therapy, Joe has regained some movement. When he returned from Hawaii, he says he "couldn't talk, sneeze, [or] laugh. I have a little more movement now from my stomach, my core. I'm still a long way from getting better."

MIKE FRITSCHNER is defying his doctors' expectations, working hard at the Kennedy Krieger Institute in Baltimore, the same center that treated actor Christopher Reeve.

Mike is determined to walk again. "At first, we started doing weight shifting, practicing balancing," he says. "And then I pretty much disregarded everything my physical therapist said and started walking. I wanted it so bad."

Mike has had to reconsider his goals. "You look at all the college entrance exams," he says. "If I'm not an athlete, what am I? How am I going to get into the school of my choice? How am I going to set myself apart from anyone else? You just work as hard as you can academically, and just hope it gets better."

Mike, now a senior, is excelling in school and running for student body president. His injury does not seem to be holding him back.

"At first, people were a little bit awkward," he says. "But if you're okay with it, then it doesn't matter to them. My friends will still come and tackle me while I'm sitting in my chair . . . in public!"

People are amazed at what Mike's been able to accomplish and they're inspired by his courage. "To be honest, I don't ever think it's a big deal," he says. "You work with whatever you've got, no matter what. You work as hard as you can. I mean, everyone I know is so close to me and supportive—my friends, family, just everyone. And my mom always told me to never give up and never say never. That's really how I live my life."

16. THE HUMAN POPSICLES

IT'S THE DEAD OF WINTER OUTSIDE THE RUBIN MUSEUM OF HIMALAYAN Art in New York City, and it's cold outside on the sidewalk, where a crowd jostles to see something almost unbelievable. Dutchman Wim Hof, a bearded man in a white terry-cloth bathrobe, is about to turn himself into a human Popsicle. While the crowd is bundled up against the cold, Hof, who was forty-eight years old when he performed this particular feat, strips down to gray shorts, gets into a glass enclosure about the size of a telephone booth, and has ice chips poured in up to his neck. It looks as though he's been planted in a snowbank—and he looks perfectly calm.

An ambulance is at the ready. Dr. Kenneth Kamler, a New York microsurgeon and author of *Surviving the Extremes: A Doctor's Journey to the Limits of Human Endurance*, a book about "extreme medicine" that tests the boundaries of what the body can do, is on hand to watch for danger signs.

"It's almost beyond belief that anyone could live through that," says Kamler. "He's not moving. He's not generating heat. He's immersed in ice water. And water will transmit heat thirty times faster than air. It literally sucks the life right out of you."

Wim is unfazed. He stays in the ice for one hour and twelve minutes—a new world record.

A CHILLY MYSTERY

Scientists can't really explain how Wim, known as "The Ice Man," is able to withstand temperatures that would kill the average person. It's an ability he discovered thirty years ago as a young man, strolling by an icy pond in a park. "I saw the ice," Wim says. "And I thought: what would happen if I go in there? I was really attracted to it. I got rid of my clothes. Thirty seconds, I was in. Tremendous good feeling when I came out. And since then, I repeated it every day."

Wim has been on a lifelong quest to push the limits of human endurance. He traveled one hundred miles north of the Arctic Circle in January to run a half marathon—in his bare feet. He swam almost twice the distance of a fifty-meter Olympic-size pool *under* the ice at the North Pole, dressed only in a swimsuit.

That was all a warm-up (forgive the pun) for his next feat—being the first person to attempt to climb Mount Everest in sandals, shorts, and a headband.

"No one has come close to climbing Everest without protection from the cold," says Kamler. "It's almost inconceivable."

While he did not summit Everest (something which he hopes to do in the future), he climbed to quite a high altitude. "It [was] quite easy," he says. "I was in a snowstorm, fifteen, sixteen, eighteen thousand feet." He says he was able to do this barely dressed because "I know my body. I know my mind."

What's going on here? Doctors are all too familiar with the usual consequences of this kind of exposure: frostbite and hypothermia are dangers when we're exposed to the kind of cold Wim routinely endures (perhaps *enjoys* would be more accurate). "Your body begins to shut down in a very selective way," Kamler says. "It diverts blood flow entirely away from areas that are not necessary for immediate survival, such as the ears, toes, fingers, nose. Your body will then do everything it can to protect the more vital functions. But if not treated immediately, the damage to those body parts is irreversible. The other danger is hypothermia. When your core body temperature drops below ninety degrees, the vital organs start shutting down. Once that starts, you could be dead within minutes."

Not Wim. Scientists are studying him to discover how he is able to survive his freezing exploits and emerge from them with no problems—no frostbite, no hypothermia—hale and hearty.

THE HIMALAYAN CONNECTION

At the University of Minnesota Hypothermia Lab, researchers wanted to know exactly what was happening to Wim's vital signs when he was exposed to dangerously low temperatures. They already know how normal people respond to freezing temperature. In one recent experiment, a British military diver was immersed in a tank filled with fifty-degree water. His reaction was immediate—intense pain, cardiovascular stress, and mounting panic.

But we watched them put Wim into even colder water. He was perfectly calm. "I feel the cold is a noble force . . . I like it."

They've taken all the baseline measurements of Wim's body—and he's completely normal physically. Doctors can't help but conclude: Wim's secret is his brain.

"It's very easy to speculate that the same mind control that you use to control your heart when you're scared also can be called upon to control the other organs in the body," says Kamler. "And maybe that's how Wim does this."

One answer might lie in a Himalayan meditation practice called Tummo that Wim began practicing years ago. It's an ancient technique developed by Tibetans and other practitioners of Himalayan Buddhism, which has, as its primary goal, the attainment of wisdom and compassion. A well-known side effect? It generates heat. Legends abound of naked Tummo practitioners who sit on ice, in freezing temperatures, draped with wet sheets. As they meditate, the sheets dry and the ice melts around them.

Wim practices breathing exercises and esoteric yoga techniques. He says his ability to withstand being submerged in ice cubes and swimming under arctic ice has to do with practicing mind control, breath control, meditation, regularly submitting himself to extremes of cold water, and being in top physical shape.

TUNING

When most people fall into cold water, they scream, shout, and thrash; their heart rate rockets; they hyperventilate. In short, they panic. Not Wim. He's psychologically prepared. "It's like turning on a button," he says, "a thermostat, and bringing in a certain kind of force, which is able to withstand the impact [of the cold]. I call it tuning. It's meditation. Ordinary people get berserk; they are out of control. Cold shock can be trained. You have to train your body. But it's absolutely the mind which is able to steer energies within the body."

Wim says he doesn't break records just for fun, or even for the publicity, but he's happy to undertake what looks impossible for a good cause: "If people ask me to do a world record, for example, do a full marathon in shorts on the North Pole, I'll do that in a way that I can raise money for charity."

With our jaws dropped, we watched Wim stroll around Duluth, Minnesota, in shorts. The weather service told us that, with the wind chill, it was negative thirteen degrees. It looks pretty physical, but Wim says he approaches his encounters with the cold as a spiritual path. "If we talk about spirituality, then that means to be able to sit and to feel really good, and to understand what God is all about and the presence of being here. And that's what I feel by immersing myself in the [cold] water."

Wim also thinks that immersion in the cold is what keeps him fit. Constricting and opening up veins can cleanse the cardiovascular system and prevent diseases, including heart disease, thrombosis, and diabetes. "The blood flow is better, people will feel better," he says. But, he cautions, "People need to extend themselves, slowly exposing themselves to cold."

_____

THE WHITE DEATH

There is some evidence that Wim isn't entirely immune to cold—he's had hypothermia when he climbed out of cold water and his core temperature dropped. Blood from the cold surface of his body mixed with the warmer blood from his core. Scientists call this the "after drop." Wim describes it as a "horrific feeling": delirium, heaviness, and pain. He felt "very strange," he says, "out of control. You're just a victim of forces. And you feel like you are going to die."

But he says during these instances of hypothermia, he was able to will himself back from the brink.

Wim also experienced hypothermia twice as a child, at ages seven and twelve. He was in the snow. Fatigue overtook him. The snow was inviting. He lay down and went to sleep in it and was brought to the hospital with hypothermia. "It's a nice fatigue," he says. "The nicest death is the white death."

Setting world records in the cold is risky. Once, Wim's retina froze while he was swimming fifty meters under the ice. "I had no goggles on," he says. "I deviated from the route. I didn't see anything. At eighty meters, my powers faded away, little by little. I didn't feel any agony. I could have swum into death. But then I felt a diver grabbing my ankle. He brought me back to the fifty-meter hole."

Wim says that when he was preparing to have ice poured onto him out on that sidewalk, he was full of energy. "I say hello to people, but, actually, I'm gone. I'm not in the world. I'm awaiting my appointment with my friend, which is cold. I think anybody, if he is driven enough, can withstand just about anything, and without pain. I repeat my goal, I see my goal, I visualize it. Sometimes it is painful if I divert toward people or let myself go a little bit. Then, suddenly, it begins to really hurt here or there. Then, I'm directing, once again, my mind toward the spot where this negative impact is going on. It takes about a minute for it to fade away."

By the way, when he swam eighty meters under the ice, Wim also held his breath for a full six minutes by regulating his respiration and heartbeat.

"We have the power to have a certain control over the heart," Wim says. "You can do that by directing the mind toward the heartbeat, and make it beat less per minute. I think if you control the mind in order not to have this trafficking of thought all the time, then you really have mastered what life is all about."

"I know my body, I know my mind, I know what I can do," he says. "Through years you learn how to handle these extremes."

Our correspondent on this segment of *Medical Mysteries*, Juju Chang, wanted to compare her reaction with Wim's in a cold water tank. She and Wim both immersed their feet.

Her immediate response: "I'm in a lot of discomfort. Oh, my God, it's painful . . ."

Wim didn't even flinch.

After just a few minutes, their dramatically different skin temperatures told the story: Chang, 81.3 degrees; Hof, 90.4.

Wim's explanation? "You have to remain in control," he says.

No matter how cold it gets, the ice man stays as cool as the proverbial cucumber.

HE'S NOT ALONE

American long-distance swimmer Lynn Cox seems to be as impervious to the cold as Wim Hof. In 2002 she traveled south to attempt the first-ever mile-long swim *in thirty-two-degree water*—among the icebergs of Antarctica.

Like Wim, Lynn uses her brain to raise her core temperature, in essence forcing her body to run a high fever.

Preparing for her swim, Lynn said she "sat down, focused, breathed, and thought about how I was going to enter the water. How I was going to do the swim. I went through a mental rehearsal of it. My body knew that I was going to jump into very cold water. Before I went in, my core temperature was 102.2. Buddhist monks can do it; maybe I can, too."

Lynn knew her teeth could shatter in the cold water. She had three coats of fluoride painted on them to protect them from the cold. She says that being only five-six and "having extra body fat to act as an internal wet suit helps."

Lynn went for her swim with a standby crew—three zodiac boats, three doctors, a diver in a dry suit, and a cowroper friend from Nebraska who could throw a lasso around her in case she couldn't get out of the water.

Wearing just a one-piece swimsuit and goggles, Lynn walked down a gangplank into the frigid Antarctic waters. "The air temperature was thirty-two degrees, and the wind was gusting at thirty-five knots," she says. "It was like stepping on ice trays as I kept coming down the stairs."

Lynn swam in thirty-two-degree water for twenty-five minutes.

"What I learned was that I could swim in water that was basically liquid ice," she says.

Should you find yourself, most likely against your will, in freezing water, Lynn, like Wim, says it's important not to panic. The best thing to do is to keep still. "For somebody falling into cold water, the general idea is that you just stay where you are," says Lynn. "You give off heat, and you actually create a little layer of warmer water around your body, which acts as [an] insulator to keep you warm. But if you move, and you're not acclimated to the cold, you're basically circulating the cool blood from the outside right into the core, and that causes your temperature to drop. I've acclimated. I spent many years doing it, and I really focus on it when I swim. I am able to vasoconstrict and stay closed down. Basically, my body is saying: if you need to, lose your hands, lose your feet, lose your arms, lose your legs, but keep your core warm."

COLD YET?

Hypothermia, teeth shattering, nerve damage, frostbite, and half-ton leopard seals—these were dangers Lynn faced on her swim. The one she didn't see coming: moving icebergs. Lynn ran into one and bumped her head. Her friend Dan joked afterward that she should ice it.

Lynn started cold-water swimming as a teenager when she found that during swim workouts in pools she would overheat. At fifteen, she started swim training in the ocean with the goal of crossing the English Channel.

Lynn has been working with scientists who are experimenting with various warming techniques. They kept tabs on her as she swam across the Bering Strait from Alaska to Russia. The scientists monitored her core temperature by having her swallow a tiny thermometer that sent out radio signals. On this long swim, through thirty-eight-degree water, Lynn's core temperature remained constant.

After her Bering swim, a Russian doctor put hot water bottles on her carotid, brachial, and femoral arteries and had her climb into a sleeping bag—the goal was to warm her slowly. This technique caused her to shiver uncontrollably and exhausted her.

She looked for other ways to warm herself up after her freezing immersions. She swam in the Canadian Arctic off Baffin Island for twenty-three minutes in 28.8 degree water, the temperature at which salt water freezes. After this swim, she put on dry clothes and a parka and walked quickly up snow-covered hills back to her hotel, where she got into a cold shower and gradually turned up the temperature of the water until it was warm. Within a half hour, her temperature was back to normal and she was able to go sightseeing. "I felt like I needed to figure out a better way to re-warm, because I didn't think that shivering was successful. I wasn't shaking for an hour, and I wasn't exhausted for the next three days," she says.

HOW THE COLD KILLS—THAT IS, WHAT WOULD HAPPEN TO YOU OR ME

Dr. Kamler describes what happens to an average body when we get chilled. "Our body temperature is 98.6, roughly," says Kamler. "And if we go more than ten degrees above or below [that], the body starts to break down. The body has mechanisms to protect you when you get cold. First, divert blood flow away from the outside part of your skin [where] it exchanges temperature with the outside environment. That's how you regulate your temperature. But when your body senses that you're cold, it diverts the blood flow away from the superficial areas of your skin, to below a layer of fat that all of us have beneath the skin. And that's sort of like tucking your toes into a blanket to keep warm. When that's not enough, your body goes to [the] next mechanism—goose bumps, the body's attempt to create loft."

The puckering of your skin in goose bumps raises the hair on your body; that's the "loft," which creates space for warm air and works very well for birds and furry mammals. "It's kind of pathetic for humans because we don't have all that much hair, and it doesn't really create much loft on your skin," Kamler notes.

When all this fails, the body begins to shiver, random muscle contractions that generate a tremendous amount of heat. If shivering doesn't warm you up, your body begins to shut down in a very selective way. It diverts blood flow entirely away from places that are superficial and are not necessary for immediate survival: that would be your ears, toes, fingers, and nose. Those places are exposed to air, and they have a very high surface area, which means they rapidly lose heat. Your body does everything it can to protect your more vital organs: heart, lungs, and brain.

"It will shut down other mechanisms, such as your immune system, your digestive system, your reproductive system," Kamler says. "You don't need those systems for immediate survival. It will shut down your higher thinking areas, [which] aren't necessary for survival."

When your body temperature reaches eighty-five degrees or so, "that's when your heart stops, and that's when it's fatal," says Kamler.

Wim's "white death."

DEFYING SCIENCE

Wim and Lynn defy medical science. And if you're waiting for us to give you the "secret" of how they do it, sorry. This one's still a mystery. "Neither one of them should be able to do what they do," Kamler says. "Yet they do it. So how do they do it? The answer to that lies deep within the brain. It's a mystery that we have not yet come close to solving, although we do have tantalizing clues."

By going where no humans have gone before, Wim Hof and Lynn Cox are giving scientists insights that might someday help the rest of us unleash the untapped power of our minds. In the meantime, they are pushing the limits of human endurance, reentering the cold again and again, drawn to it in the same way flowers are drawn to the sun.

And I'm going to put on an extra pair of socks now.

17. REVERSED ORGANS

Y OU'VE READ ABOUT SOME UNUSUAL MEDICAL CASES IN THIS BOOK: strange allergies, odd genetic disorders, and bizarre and inexplicable behaviors in otherwise perfectly healthy people. But in none of the medical mysteries we investigated did we come up with a stranger condition than the one afflicting the two girls you'll learn about below. They look perfectly normal on the outside. Inside is another story.

It's a condition that isn't as rare as you might think. One in ten thousand people are born with it, and you'll probably be as incredulous as we were when we first heard about it.

KAY SALOMON

When we interviewed her for the show, Kay Salomon was by all appearances, and against all odds, a strapping nine-year-old girl who loved soccer and skateboarding. Kay's good health amazed her mother, Kerry McCauley: doctors had handed Kay a death sentence when she was a newborn.

Two days after her birth, doctors detected a murmur in Kay's heart. That was cause for concern, but many babies have heart murmurs. On further investigation, doctors found that Kay had what's called "corrected transposition": the right atrium of her heart was on the left side; the left atrium on the right side. Her ventricles were where they were supposed to be, but her aorta came off her right ventricle, and her pulmonary artery came off her left ventricle. In other words, they were reversed as well.

The doctors at Miami Children's Hospital told Kerry that Kay's condition was extremely rare; they'd only read about it. Never seen it. And then they told Kerry that not only did her daughter have an extremely rare heart defect, she had something else almost as frightening: asplenia syndrome—she had been born without a spleen.

An adult can live without a spleen. But not a child. It serves a vital immune function—and a child's immune system is more easily overwhelmed by infection.

DON'T BELIEVE EVERYTHING YOU HEAR

Kerry left the hospital with an oral prescription for antibiotics for Kay. She was told Kay would need to take antibiotics for the rest of her life to keep her from developing any kind of bacterial infection, which, without a protective spleen, could be fatal.

But Kerry couldn't accept this dire prognosis. Though the doctors said a missing spleen was related to Kay's heart condition, it didn't make sense to Kerry. "I want [a] test," she remembers insisting. "I don't believe it." To which the doctor replied: "Don't disappoint yourself. It's 99.9 percent." No spleen. No future.

"I started traveling around the country with Kay—she was eight months old—looking for answers. I took her to St. Mary's Children's Hospital in West Palm Beach for an abdomen ultrasound to look for a spleen. They told me: 'Sorry, [no] spleen.' I kept searching. I just didn't want to believe."

Finally, when Kerry took Kay for a renal ultrasound at West Boca Hospital, the test turned up a remarkable result. It confirmed what Kerry had intuitively felt. Kay did have a spleen—it was just on the wrong side of her body. In fact, Kerry learned, *all* Kay's organs were reversed—everything inside her was on the opposite side of her body from where it is in the rest of us! This is generally a genetic condition.

"I jumped up with joy!" Kerry says. "[I] was so happy that Kay had a spleen."

A PRECARIOUS BALANCE

The complete organ reversal on top of her heart condition made Kay's case extremely rare.

"We thought it was one in a million," says Kerry. "It's probably rarer than that."

It was amazing that, with all the reversed organs, Kay's body was working as well as it was. Most of her "backwards" organs wouldn't cause any problems, but her heart's reversal carried an extra threat. Because the arteries and veins are "backwards," Kay's heart could give out at any time. This keeps her mother in a state of almost constant anxiety—hovering over her daughter in the night while she's sleeping, watching every breath. "I go in there many times during the night and check on her to make sure she's okay, because it could happen, it might not happen, but nobody knows."

The upper chambers and major arteries in Kay's heart are switched, yet, amazingly, her blood still goes where it's supposed to go—it's just using all the wrong connections.

Dr. Frank Hanley, a pediatric cardiac surgeon at Packard Children's Hospital in California, says: "The easy way to look at that is 'two wrongs make it right.'" He isn't worried so much about the unique structure of Kay's heart, but about the fact that she has a large hole between the lower chambers and an obstruction under one of her valves.

"Most of the time, if you have only one of those, you have to have surgery relatively early in life," Hanley says.

But Kay, at nine, seems to be functioning well. "Her circulation, as we say in the business, is perfectly balanced," says Hanley.

That balance, unfortunately, is a precarious one. Specialists have told Kerry that people with similar defects often wear out their hearts and die before they reach the age of forty.

"Here's a little girl who's perfectly fine right now," says Hanley. "But you could make the argument that there's never a better time to do the procedure because this is when her heart is the healthiest. Whether we can wait five years, ten years, and get the same result with the same low risk, it's hard to say."

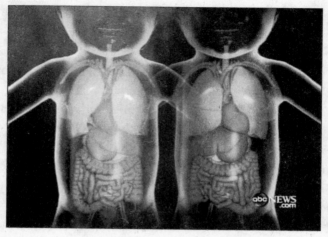

Left: Normal organ placement.
Right: Reversed organ placement.

A COMPLICATED SURGERY

The "procedure" to which Hanley refers is open-heart surgery. Because of the mix-up in Kay's heart, her smaller, weaker heart valve is responsible for pumping blood to the entire body, rather than just the lungs as it would in a "frontways" heart. The valve could give out. But waiting could make an operation more difficult than it already is. Maybe impossible.

Dr. Ira Parnass, a top cardiologist at Mount Sinai Hospital in New York City, has been following Kay's case.

Kay is "the rarest of the rare," he says. He describes the operation that would fix her heart: "We can switch the atria. We can run complicated baffles, they're called, to do that switch. Then we can do an arterial switch of some sort. We can resect the obstruction under the pulmonary artery. And we can close the ventricular septal defect. We can do all that. But we can't do it at no risk."

On average, three out of one hundred patients in Kay's position die from the surgery she needs. That sounds like good odds, unless it's your child. And what if the child, like Kay, seems just fine and is leading a normal life?

Kerry says most of the surgeons with whom she's consulted have serious reservations about doing such a complicated operation. "They don't want to tell me what to do," says Kerry, "because it's just so complex. Most surgeons say to leave her alone. I brought her to Duke, and their team said they're against it. I brought her to Children['s Hospital in] Boston, and they were against it. I brought her to UCLA, and [they] said that she might be better off left alone."

"I always tell patients [that] statistics lie with respect to an individual," says Parness. "You either escape the complication or not. So now the question is, are you so convinced you need to do this that in the awful, unlikely possibility that she doesn't make it through the surgery and she dies, you can live with that decision?"

Kerry says the choice—to operate or not to operate—is driving her mad. "It's the worst decision for me possibly to try to make. And it's causing me such stress. I sleep with it, I wake up with nightmares and anxiety attacks. Thinking, 'Am I doing the right thing, [to] leave her alone?'"

Kerry has been in touch with another family whose daughter, only a year younger than Kay, has a similarly shaped heart, but without Kay's additional complication of reversed organs. They have been helping Kerry weigh the odds and giving her hope that even if she and Kay decide the operation is necessary, everything will turn out fine.

CARLEY PRESTON

The Prestons are that other family—dealing, in their home in Ohio, with many of the same issues as Kerry and Kay.

Like Kay, their daughter Carley appeared to be a perfectly healthy pink-skinned newborn.

"She looked perfectly fine," says her mother, Tanya. "But the test results [said] she should be critical. In dire straits."

Carley was rushed to Rainbow Babies, a children's hospital in Cleveland.

Doctors found that Carley's heart was reversed in much the same way as Kay's. But in Carley's case there was a significant obstruction in the artery that carried blood to her lungs.

Doctors told the Prestons that Carley would need an operation by age four. As she grew, the Prestons sought second, third, and fourth opinions.

It was Tanya who brought the two families together—she read an article about Kay and felt, mom to mom, that she had to call Kerry.

"I mean, friends are nice and supportive but until you've been there . . . ," she says.

So now the two families are a support network for each other, and Kerry has been closely following Carley's progress. Carley's obstruction in her lung artery meant that her body wasn't getting enough oxygenated blood from the lungs. Unlike Kay, she couldn't run as fast or for as long as her peers, and she was often what doctors call "blue," a term that refers to the skin color of someone whose heart isn't working right.

Tanya remembers explaining to Carley that her heart was different. "She had just assumed that everyone had heart defects," Tanya says. "It never crossed her mind that she was any different. I was tucking her in bed one night and she asked me what *my* heart defects were. Which ones I had." Tanya told her daughter she didn't have any defects. "Well, what about Daddy?" Carley asked. "Which ones does Daddy have?" "Daddy doesn't have any either," said Tanya. "She ran through her sisters, both sisters, she moved on to grandparents. And after grandparents, she started to move to aunts and uncles. At this point, she says—'Wait a minute. I'm the only one?' That never crossed her mind, which I found humorous. She's grown up in knowing it makes you special, but you don't get special treatment because of it. Your sisters can still pick on you if you have it coming. She's grown up normal. She feels no different."

Tanya is able to find humor in the story now—after deciding that Carley should have the surgery. The Prestons took the plunge because they saw that Carley's quality of life was suffering. They waited until she was seven years old—and doctors told them their little girl's oxygen levels were dropping. Tanya felt "elated" when they finally made the decision to go ahead. Elated and relieved; she was exhausted by the daily merry-go-round: "what to do and when to do it."

The operation took nearly five hours; surgeons worked to reroute Carley's "backwards" blood flow to mimic a normal heart. A bypass machine took over pumping her blood while her problematic valve was replaced with an artificial one. The surgery was so taxing that Carley was kept under anesthesia for two days after the operation so her heart could rest.

Tanya remembers how beautiful her daughter looked after the operation—even though she was still anesthetized.

"You could immediately see a difference in her," says Tom. "In her color and her face and so forth. But it was nerve-racking to see your child laying in the, in the hospital room, all the lines going into her."

But Carley made a quick recovery. Just four weeks after surgery, she was able to go on a five-mile bike ride and climb an incline, which she had never been able to do without stopping to rest.

"It was absolutely amazing," says Tom. "A proud moment."

Since the operation, Carley has been a completely normal, active, healthy girl. The only sign of her condition is a red dot and a faint line down the middle of her chest where the surgeon made his incision.

"I don't really care about it; in the summers I just wear swimsuits that cover up my scar. But all my friends know, so it doesn't really matter to me or them. I just have one big bump. [People] just think it's an infected mosquito bite or something."

Carley will need to get a valve replacement when she is in middle school.

"Future operations are required because children outgrow valves that are put in, just like they outgrow their T-shirts and shoes," says Hanley.

With modern medicine on her side, Carley is likely to live a normal life span. It's something Kerry McCauley dreams of for Kay.

For now, however, Kay is a true medical mystery, a little girl whose insides are so wrong but work together just right—"backwards."

The question remains—for how long? It's a question that haunts her mother day and night.

18. "CURIOUSER AND CURIOUSER"

REMEMBER *ALICE'S ADVENTURES IN WONDERLAND*? ALICE FALLS down the rabbit hole. She finds a bottle on a table labeled, "Drink Me," downs the contents, and shrinks to the size of a mouse. She then spies a piece of cake with the words "Eat Me." She takes a bite and grows gigantically tall.

What if this particular part of Alice's adventures wasn't just a fairy tale? What if it was an all too real medical mystery?

ALL IN THE FAMILY

Katie O'Brien, nineteen when we interviewed her, often feels like Alice at the bottom of the rabbit hole. Katie's reality can change in the blink of an eye.

"It usually happens early in the morning," Katie says. "Right when I wake up."

Katie can open her eyes to a world that has shrunk to the proportions of a dollhouse: everyday objects, strangely tiny. On other mornings, she wakes to a world that is weirdly large.

"I was looking at the couch once and it looked like the couch was growing," she says. "That was really weird. Really horrible."

As a little girl, Katie says she wasn't frightened by these odd shifts in perception: "It was just something that didn't make sense. Something I didn't understand."

Katie's mother, Denise, sympathized. She says she had the same bizarre experiences as a child: "I just remember feeling really tiny and everything got really big. And, then it reverses. It's a *very* odd sensation."

Denise was in her twenties before she had any explanation for these hallucinogenic episodes, which, in both mother and daughter, last for about thirty minutes. Denise discovered that she and now her daughter share a rare condition called Alice in Wonderland syndrome, named, of course, after Alice's adventures. Alice describes her symptoms in the book: " 'Now I'm opening out like the largest telescope that ever was. Good-bye, feet.' For when she looked down at her feet, they seemed to be almost out of sight."

KATIE'S SISTER, Molly, doesn't grow or shrink. For her, "I get what I always called fast-and-slow. I remember one time I was in the bathtub, and the dripping water sounded really, really fast. It wasn't distorted—it was just really, really fast. Other times, people would be talking on TV, and they'd be talking really, really slow."

Besides these odd perceptions, the women in the O'Brien family share another family trait—migraines. They are three of roughly 28 million Americans who suffer from them.

Alice in Wonderland syndrome, the O'Briens' odd visual and auditory experiences, are part of what doctors call an "aura." That's a set of perceptions that happen before the on-set of a migraine and can also presage a seizure (remember our chapter on Stacey Gayle, the girl whose aura, strange smells, preceded her music seizures).

Auras are one of the things that distinguish a migraine from a really bad headache. Molly's dramatic time displacement "aura" tells her a migraine is on the way. She also sees multiple images of the letter C that look like "thousands of little sequins, iridescent colored sequins, all overlapping. They're circular. There's no angle—no shards of glass. They shimmer, but they're all different colors. They're flat. They sparkle different colors—blues, greens, and pinks—shimmer and pop. It's like a flashbulb. It stays when you close your eyes. It's very bright. It'll be dark on the outside, but it'll still be there, and it'll still shimmer and shine."

AURAS AND MIGRAINE

The Mayo Clinic's Dr. David Dotick, an expert in migraines and their accompanying auras, says those strange altera-tions in perception or physical sensations that the O'Brien girls experience are typical of migraine sufferers who have auras. "The sense of the feet seeming to get so far away is rather typical, actually, of the patients who describe this sort of distortion of the body image," says Dotick.

Molly's vivid shimmering field of C's? Also typical.

"Sometimes patients describe mosaic vision, where they see a picture or your face that's fractured and looks like it's in little pieces," Dotick says. "Or zoom vision, where things seem very, very far away or very, very close."

Some people feel as though only a part of their body is morphing. One patient of Dotick's said it was as if her ear were ballooning out six inches.

And who knows how many people have Alice in Wonderland and never say a word about it? Migraine sufferers, Dotick says, "think they're going crazy. And that's why they tend not to share it. I think it's probably more common than we now recognize."

He estimates that migraine aura itself occurs in 15 to 20 percent of people with migraine. "You do the math," he says. "That's a lot of people that could be afflicted with migraine aura."

Millions of people.

Auras and the migraines that follow can be triggered spontaneously in genetically susceptible patients. Migraines often run in families, as is the case with the O'Briens. Again, Dotick suggests this isn't as widely recognized, even by migraine sufferers, as it should be. He always asks his patients if they have a family history of migraine. Many say no. But after Dotick probes, he often uncovers a mother who went to bed sick with headaches or a father who suffered from what he called "sinus" headaches, which were actually migraines, Dotick suggests. "Patients who tell me they don't have a family history—I usually say: 'We need to go back and dig deeper in your family. I'm sure it's there somewhere.'"

There are many different types of migraines (some, oddly, in other parts of the body and some without pain), but the most common migraine is a severe headache, often accompanied by nausea, without the Alice auras that Katie and Denise experience.

In one type of migraine attack, genes have been identified that affect chemical pathways into the cells. When too much of some chemicals get in, the cells "short circuit," says Dotick. "It's kinda like a short circuit in the brain, that's genetically predetermined, and it will create this sort of burst of activity and that will spread across the brain. And it will do so at a very slow rate. Maybe three millimeters per minute. Which is why these visual illusions sort of evolve over a period of time. It takes time to travel over the brain."

Auras don't necessarily mean you'll have a headache. "You tell them they have migraine aura, and they immediately say no, I didn't have a headache," says Dotick. "Everybody thinks that if you have migraine you must have headaches."

ALICE'S ADVENTURES IN IMAGING

Back to Katie O'Brien. She says the migraines that follow her Alice auras are excruciatingly painful. "Like knives in your head, it's horrible stuff." Aspirin and other pain relievers don't seem to help. The way she gets through the migraines is by sleeping. "I think that's the only thing I've ever been able to do that's gotten rid of it is just go to sleep," she says.

It helps if she's in a dark room with no sound.

Scholars speculate that Lewis Carroll, whose real name was Charles Dodgson, a mathematics professor at Oxford University, may have suffered from migraine auras when he wrote *Alice's Adventures in Wonderland*. He created the story for ten-year-old Alice Liddell, thought to be the real Alice.

Dotick says he is no Carroll scholar, but he knows that people interested in both literature and neurology have examined Carroll's life and work. "The question is whether he suffered from migraine aura when he was doing his writing because he hadn't recorded that in his diaries," Dotick says. "But there's no question that he did suffer from aura" at some point.

It would be 150 years after Carroll penned *Alice* before science would begin to unravel the mystery of why auras such as Katie's occur.

At Seattle Radiologists, researchers are attempting to capture, for the first time, an actual picture of Alice in Wonderland syndrome in the brain of twelve-year-old Ana Ryseff. Ana, who lives in Seattle, was diagnosed in the third grade. Her auras last just a few minutes and only seem to happen when she's concentrating hard on a printed page.

"Sometimes when I'm really focusing on a piano piece, the notes will just zoom up. So they're just really big, like, as if you were using a camera and you zoomed up on someone."

At other times, the size of the entire sheet of music will blow up in front of her. The same thing can happen when she's reading. "I'm just looking at the book, holding it. My hands are the same size, but the book expands—everything on the book, the pages, words, just everything. I was thinking: What the heck is happening? I had no clue."

If you'd like a little dose of irony, what part did Ana get in the school play? Alice.

Kim Ryseff, Ana's mother, a teacher, says that these auras scared her daughter when she was little. "She would cry out in the night. We often laid down with her and she would say, 'Mommy, everything is getting really big in the room.' The first couple of times we were tired and said, 'Yeah, yeah. Uh-huh.' We kind of ignored it. Probably the third time we realized this was something a little unusual. We weren't really concerned. Because my husband seemed to remember having something similar happen to him when he was younger."

Eventually, however, as the aura persisted Ana's pediatrician sent the Ryseffs to a neurologist and Ana ended up with a diagnosis: Alice in Wonderland syndrome.

Neurologist Dr. Sheena Aurora had a hunch he could trigger Ana's aura inside a scanner and get a functional image of her brain. Researchers used a flashing black-and-white checkerboard pattern to mimic the black and white of the printed page. They had Ana focus on a little dot and watched as an aura took over her vision. Usually when someone sees something, the part of the brain that processes images "lights up" on the screen. What is remarkable is that in the back of Ana's brain, *two* areas fire at once. A burst of electrical activity causes abnormal blood flow in the area that processes vision—and also in the part of the brain that processes texture, size, and shape.

Aurora says that those two areas of the brain lighting up "definitely can explain the differences in size and shape and form."

One of the reasons that Aurora is so interested in auras is because he, too, has them, along with their dreaded counterpart—migraine headache. He has volunteered himself as a subject in his own lab. Here's a description from the guinea pig himself: "A scintillating scotoma. Bright jagged lines that start in one part of my vision and then grow slowly. It leaves behind a black spot where I can't see anything. Then I see little shiny white and bright zigzag lines. I have pretty much the classic textbook migraine with aura. When we first started [these] experiments, I volunteered to have them done [on] myself so I knew what my subjects were going to go through."

Aurora says that after five or six minutes of looking at a black-and-white checkerboard pattern, the aura appeared. The scanner showed that more than just his visual or occipital cortex was active.

"The activity just exploded," he says. "It spread to the higher visual cortexes and also the part of the brain that's not involved with vision at all, like the parietal area."

This activity throughout the brain could account for Aurora's strange perceptions and sensations.

WHEN WE INTERVIEWED HER, Ana said she had been getting auras about once a week, when she was reading or playing the piano. The black and white of the piano's keys seemed to be a visual trigger for Alice to pay a visit, as well as the black letters on a white page.

Aurora has told Ana not to despair. Like Alice in Wonderland, Ana's adventures will likely have a happy ending. The Alice syndrome tends to disappear as the patient ages. It's already slipping away from Katie. And for Denise, it's just a memory, a looking glass version of reality.

What a relief! And as Alice herself would have said, no longer "curiouser and curiouser."

19. SEA LEGS

M OST PEOPLE KNOW WHAT IT'S LIKE TO NOT HAVE THEIR SEA legs on a choppy boat ride, or to feel queasy on a bumpy plane trip. But what if you felt like that *all the time*—if, right now as you sit still in a chair and read this, you felt the ground swaying beneath you? And the only relief from it—and this is the real twist—was to get back onto something that's moving, a boat or plane or car? It's a pretty bizarre fate: feeling like you're on the deck of a rolling ship, and you can never get off.

It's a rare disorder called disembarkment syndrome, a case of the brain learning something, then never letting it go.

DIVA-LICIOUS

A free cruise! It sounded great to Kimberly Johnson, who lived in Delray Beach, Florida. Three days and four nights off the coasts of the Bahamas in September 2002, and her mother's company was paying for it! Sure enough, Kimberly and her mother and siblings had a splendid time on *The Majesty of the Seas:* snorkeling, sunbathing, dining, drinking, and dancing. Kimberly felt lucky: the world was her oyster. She describes herself as a "princess. I was diva-licious, to say the least."

During the cruise she was constantly aware of the movement of the boat, especially when she was in her cabin: "I would say to everyone, 'Do you feel that? Can you feel the boat moving?' And they never felt anything. When I got off, my world was turned upside down."

The Majesty of the Seas returned to the Port of Miami, and Kimberly and her family disembarked. But, in a way, Kimberly did not—she continued to feel the motion of the ocean. It was as though she were still cruising in the Bahamas—and it wasn't a pleasant feeling. She says her world kept moving, "shifting back and forth, left to right. Sometimes even up and down, like a seesaw."

The feeling persisted, and Kimberly teetered through her days—queasy at least, sometimes downright nauseated—a case of seasickness on dry land that just wouldn't go away. She finally went to see her doctor.

"He kind of laughed at me and said, 'It'll go away,'" says Kimberly. "'It's just your sea legs. You've been on a cruise.'" He thought she might have vertigo and prescribed meclizine and a steroid called prednisone. Kimberly gained fifteen pounds in two weeks. The meclizine made her tired. And worse, the medications weren't working; she still felt as though she were rocking and bobbing, even when she was sitting still. The constant queasiness and dizziness were exhausting. She consulted another doctor, who thought she might have a brain tumor. A battery of tests, including an MRI, came back normal. Her doctors were baffled.

Kimberly felt her every moment had been taken over by her condition. "Everything is moving. The walls are moving.

The doors are moving. Pictures are moving. Everything's rocking as it would on a boat, back and forth, side to side, all day long until I go to bed. It's just like being on a boat every day, all day. In five-foot seas. Ten-foot seas it feels like sometimes."

And Kimberly was stuck with it—and two years passed until she came across a doctor who had seen a few cases like hers and was able to make the diagnosis: *mal de debarquement* (MDD). Named by the French physician who initially identified it, we know it as "disembarkment syndrome." Kimberly was delighted to have a diagnosis; less delighted when she was told that there was no cure for the condition, and that it might be with her for the rest of her life.

UNABLE TO UNLEARN

Dr. Richard Lewis of the Harvard and Massachusetts Eye and Ear Infirmary says that medicine doesn't really know what causes the syndrome. Everybody has a natural tendency toward motion sickness, it's a primitive response to rapid or unusual movement. But some people get carsick driving a few blocks to the grocery store. There's a huge spectrum of response.

"I would suggest that this is not really a disease per se," says Lewis. "It's an extension of a normal response, because we all feel it when we get off a boat. But for some reason people [with MDD] feel it much longer."

People with MDD report that their symptoms are more intense when they're stationary. When they get *back* on a boat, or even drive around in a car, their world stops moving.

"When you get back on the boat, the symptoms tend to go away because you're reentering the state that you've adapted to," says Lewis. "Essentially, the brain has learned something it cannot unlearn."

It's intriguing that self-generated movement will not trigger MDD. If you run a five-hour marathon, when you stop you won't feel the motion of running. But if you're on a boat for five hours, you may still feel the motion of the boat once you disembark.

Lewis explains the why. It seems to have to do with control and anticipation. "If you're on a boat and you hit a wave and everything tilts, unless you're looking out the window, you have no idea that this is occurring," he says. "When you're moving *yourself*, if you're running, your brain is actually generating the motion. And your brain actually has access to the information and what we would call a 'motor command' that moves your body. In a car, people are usually much more symptomatic when they're *not* driving, even if they're in the front seat. Everything's the same, but they are not controlling the car. When you're controlling the car, at least indirectly, you can predict what's happening. You're turning the steering wheel; you're putting on the brake. If you're a passenger, you have no idea what's happening and it's harder for you to synthesize all this information."

Lewis says that to make the disembarkment syndrome diagnosis, the usual criterion is that the patient has to experience the feeling of motion sickness for at least one month. "It's considered a very unusual syndrome. I think it's something that's probably underdiagnosed or misdiagnosed frequently," he adds.

DRIVING, CHILDREN, AND PRAYER

Kimberly says her MDD symptoms are usually less noticeable in the morning and get worse as the day progresses. By five o'clock in the afternoon, she's often a wreck. Her husband, Jeff, is a great source of support. She told him when she met him that she was "dizzy." He didn't really understand what she was talking about, but as they dated he saw how pervasive and incapacitating her syndrome was.

"Can you deal with me being a little bit grumpier and me needing more rest and me not being able to do things?" Kim asked him.

The answer was yes.

"He's just a wonderful man, and he loves me," she says. "He's willing to take care of me. Which is nice."

Not only does Kim have Jeff, she has faith.

"My faith in God is what pushes me through," she says.

Kimberly goes to church and knows "that there [are] people out there that have it a lot worse, and that I am fortunate to have what I have. I just can't go to bed and be in a ball and cry all day and feel sorry for myself, because I just have to keep doing."

Prayer is important to her. "It helps me feel better," she says. "It gives me some sort of peace."

Kim says exercising on her treadmill helps her symptoms, as well as "no stress, and sleeping a lot."

She also says driving relieves her symptoms. As Lewis noted, MDD sufferers feel better when they're in motion.

"Driving is very important," says Kim. "But it's an evil as well as a good. When you drive, you feel great. Then you get out of the car. It's almost a curse because you feel worse, but it's so good while it lasts."

Kim's symptoms have been gradually diminishing over time, and she is hopeful that science will eventually find her a cure. She also thinks that once she has children something may shift in her that will make life easier.

"I have this theory that when we decide to have children, that maybe will cure it. I'll be normal again." She laughs. "Which will be great!"

DEB RUSSO

Kim and Deb Russo met at Harvard and Massachusetts Eye and Ear Infirmary, where Lewis is one of a small group of doctors studying this strange condition. Deb is the technology specialist at a magnet school in Springfield, Massachusetts. She, like Kimberly, contracted MDD while she was on vacation.

In April of 2004, Deb and her husband, Michael, flew to Aruba via Puerto Rico. As they took off on the last leg of the trip, their plane's flap lights flashed on, so they returned to the airport. This happened four times. Finally, a new plane was brought in, and they made it to Aruba.

Deb says that it was this flight that brought on her MDD. She did have the dream vacation she and her husband had waited for. They walked everywhere, relaxed, and had a great room on the top floor of their hotel, overlooking the ocean.

It would have been perfect. Except . . .

"I felt that the street was coming up to hit me in the face," says Deb. "Everything was rocking. It, basically, has not

stopped since. It started off as a great trip. But it ended up being a trip to hell."

Deb says she now lives much of her life feeling as though
she's "sitting out on a buoy in Boston Harbor in the middle of
the winter and there is a nor'easter coming through."

Deb, like Kim, went from doctor to doctor before her
syndrome was finally diagnosed. And when she was finally
told she had MDD, she says she, too, was told there was no
treatment for it.

"They say that this doesn't kill you but it certainly takes
your life away," says Deb. "It took my life. The life that I
knew. My husband—it's put a huge burden on him. I mean,
he does everything now. My heart breaks every day for
that."

At night, Michael's embrace is the only thing that helps
Deb control the rocking motion that haunts her days. She
says he holds her until she falls asleep. "He's an angel," Deb
says simply.

"It's not on me: it's on her," says Michael. "She's the one
suffering."

Her symptoms create "a tremendous amount of anxiety"
for Deb. "I do breathing exercises," she says. "People say that
if you can relax yourself, that will help. I've gone through
hypnosis. I pray, over and over. I've been working with an
acupuncturist for about a year. That gives me a little bit of
relief. I've also tried a number of different medications that
have been aimed at migraines."

The literature on MDD suggests that it eventually goes
away. Ten years seems to be its outside limit. It tends to occur
in middle-aged women, and often in women who suffer from
migraines. Why it seems to be so largely skewed toward

middle-aged women is something that isn't well understood, although in Deb's support group for MDD there are also two men, ages twenty-one and thirty-four.

STANDARD TREATMENT—OR LACK THEREOF

Dr. Lewis has been treating MDD with vestibular physical therapy, where people are exposed to motion. "The idea is that we can try to habituate it," he says. "Habituation means that if you expose someone to the same motion repeatedly, their responses diminish over time."

The second approach is pharmaceutical. "These don't work tremendously well," Lewis says, "but we sometimes use drugs that inhibit the balance system in the brain. Those drugs tend to be in the category [of] benzodiazapines. Valium is the best known." Unfortunately, this class of drugs is addictive, "so we don't usually like to have people on those for a long time," says Lewis. "Sometimes we use certain kinds of seizure drugs like gabapentin, which has an effect on the balance part of the brain. It tends to discharge or reduce the brain's ability to promote or prolong the response to motion. I'd say it's a mixed bag. Some people do well; some people, the drugs don't affect them at all."

Deb shares Kim's positive reaction to driving. "My younger son and I had a great conversation in the car, because in the car I'm a normal person," says Deb. "And he just said that was so nice, to have a conversation like that."

EXPERIMENTAL TREATMENTS

Desperate to know more and perhaps find relief, Deb and Kim take part in experiments designed to help them. Dr. Conrad Wall, who works with Dr. Lewis at Harvard and Massachusetts Eye and Ear Infirmary, uses a balance testing apparatus. It feeds data to a computer and measures the subject's ability to compensate while standing on a moving platform.

We put our correspondent on the platform, and his results were normal: as the platform shifted, he could keep his balance with no problems. But when Kim closed her eyes and tried to stand still for fifteen seconds, the computer measured her complete inability to control her balance.

Then came the technological wonder: a biofeedback vest Dr. Wall developed. When Kim's body tilts off center, the vest vibrates on one side or the other to tell her to straighten up. Kim's vest does seem to gradually be helping her keep her balance on the moving platform. "Pretty amazing," she comments. "I definitely felt it. It was a big improvement."

The vest is expensive and still in its experimental stage. Wall is working to make it an affordable and practical balance aid.

Meanwhile, Deb practices walking with Dr. Lars Oddsson from Boston University's NeuroMuscular Research Center, who's developing a pair of biofeedback socks embedded with pressure sensors. When her weight shifts too far to one side, the socks vibrate, a signal for her to correct her balance.

"Maybe there's hope. Maybe there's hope for somebody. Yeah!" says the indefatigable Kim. "Never thought I would be a medical mystery, but I guess I am."

In a strange way, Kim feels there is a positive aspect to disembarkment syndrome—it may have made her physical self wobbly, but it's given her inner self a new sense of poise. She says her own disability has made her much more tolerant: "It taught me to treat everyone with respect. Somebody might be serving you in a restaurant, and they might not be the nicest, but you know what? Maybe they're having a bad day. Maybe they don't feel good. Maybe there's things going on in their life that you don't know about."

If you're at all like the people who worked on Kimberly and Deb's story, you come away with a new appreciation of a simple joy: stillness. And we hope that as medicine maps more of this puzzling syndrome, its victims will be able to find what we all take for granted: peace.

20. MIDNIGHT FEAST

THEY WAKE UP IN THE MORNING WITH CRUMBS ALL OVER THEIR faces, find a trail of food and candy wrappers from the kitchen to the bedroom, and have no clue that they've been gorging themselves on junk food in the middle of the night. They have been known to eat buttered cigarettes or break their teeth on frozen pizza. They've put coffee grounds, Coca-Cola, and eggshells in a blender for a hideous tasting smoothie. When you try to wake them, they become belligerent and push you aside on their beeline to the fridge. They will not be denied. And they are fast asleep.

We've shown you people who have sex and become violent in their sleep; welcome to another bizarre and mysterious parasomnia.

Who are sleep eaters? Well, if you aren't one of them yourself, you may well know someone who is. Doctors estimate that over a million Americans, most of them women between the ages of twenty and fifty, have sleep-related eating disorder (SRED). And doctors have no idea what causes it.

AMY KOECHLER

There may be a genetic link to SRED. Amy Koechler, a teacher, may have inherited sleep eating from her mother, Shirley, who also eats in her sleep. Ever since she could toddle, Amy has been getting up in the middle of the night. Her eyes are open, and she is able to navigate through the house, walk downstairs, and, most importantly, open the kitchen cabinets and refrigerator. But by all medical measures, she is asleep, unconscious of her surroundings.

"I would get up in the middle of the night and I would grab Girl Scout cookies or a glass of juice," says Amy. "I would get my mom, and I'd pretend to have a little tea party. She became very frustrated with me because I would constantly wake her up. I was probably seven years old at that time."

Her mother quickly grew tired of the nocturnal tea parties. And her daughter wasn't always so genteel. *Gone with the Wind* could quickly start to resemble *Night of the Living Dead*.

"She would come up the stairs, and she would flop her feet like a duck," Shirley recalls. "We knew she was sleepwalking. And then she'd have these *eyes*. And you know she's not awake. Once in a while, she'd turn around and give you that evil look. And she'd scream, 'I'M HUNGRY!'"

But hunger isn't really much of a factor in sleep eating. Those afflicted have tried eating huge dinners right before bedtime; they still arise in the dead of night and head for the kitchen. Nor does sleep eating kill one's appetite in the morning. After a full night of gorging—for Amy, perhaps *eight* or *nine* trips to the fridge—she's still ready for breakfast.

Amy, as is typical with sleep eaters, tends to pack in the calories at night. "Junk foods stay in your mouth longer," she says. "Like, the chocolate; it coats your mouth. Ice cream stays in your taste buds. Versus a granola bar or a banana. You eat it, and it's gone."

Amy noticed a pattern to her sleep eating, even when she was young. She took more trips to the refrigerator in the middle of the night when she was under stress. "Days before tests or if I had a boyfriend, or if there were school dances or things with girlfriends, any type of stressful situation—my sleep eating and sleepwalking would definitely increase."

In just about all cases, sleepwalking is part of sleep eating; Amy recounts waking up on the couch with Doritos all around her and no idea how she got there. In other instances, people wake up with their bed full of food.

Amy's fiancé, Ryan, has tried hiding food—to no avail. As is the case with most sleep eaters, Amy is wily and persistent. "He's not very sneaky about it," says Amy. "I'll make some cupcakes or whatever, and he'll hide them on top of the refrigerator. But it's not a very good hiding spot."

Dreaming about eating can be part of sleep eating. Amy says she was nervous the night before the first day of her teaching internship in Eau Claire, Wisconsin. The result of this stress? An empty Cheetos bag—in the shower.

Amy says that she was dreaming that she arose in the middle of the night, thinking it was time to get ready to appear in her new role in front of a class for the first time.

"I thought it was time to get going," she says. "And I had a bag of Cheetos [that] I started eating. I had my Cheetos, and I went in the shower and started showering. Then I woke up, and I vividly remember being freezing, standing in front of my fan. I look at the clock and it's two in the morning."

Amy went back to bed. The next thing she knew—her alarm clock went off. She went to take another shower. "I want to be nice and clean for my first day of intern teaching," she recalls. "And when I step in there, there are Cheetos [in] the bottom of the shower."

It was perplexing for Amy, to say the least. She was dreaming something she had actually done. In this case, the dream and the reality were one and the same.

NO JUDGMENT, NO INHIBITION

Dr. Carlos Schenck, a leading researcher in the field of sleep medicine and codirector of the Minnesota Regional Sleep Disorders Center, has treated hundreds of sleep eaters. He says that the disorder is a "mixture of two basic instincts: sleeping and eating. When they become intertwined in a pathological way, you have this syndrome that persists night after night, for years on end, until the patients come for help."

Schenck says in this sense sleep eating is very much like sexsomnia—two basic human needs and instincts that somehow become intertwined without the patient's volition. Occasionally, he'll see sexsomnia and sleep eating in the same patient. Often, a patient with sleep eating will also have other types of sleep disorders: restless leg syndrome (an irresistible urge to move one's legs), sleepwalking, and sleep apnea.

"Most of these patients have some awareness of what they're doing," he says. "Others have no awareness. They're like sleeping zombies, walking around headless. There's a compulsion to eat. But it's not a hunger-driven behavior. Some of these people will have a complete second dinner before they go to bed at night, to suppress the urge to eat. It does not work. These people really feel compelled to eat despite not feeling hungry. The part of the brain that's asleep is the one that has the shut-down on the frontal lobes, probably, which is the seat of judgment. These people do not have proper judgment. They can get up; they see their environment. They know where the kitchen is. But they have no judgment, no inhibition. And that's the problem."

Schenck says that often his patients are shocked when they see themselves on the videotapes that Schenck makes in his clinic and in their homes. " 'My God, I didn't realize I was capable of doing this,' " Schenck says his patients often tell him. " 'How can I be asleep and do all this? It's disgusting. It's gross. It's terrible.' "

Schenck says eating when you're asleep has nothing to do with will power. "It's not a psychological problem," he says. "It's a major physiological force coming from within your brain and body to eat at night so inappropriately."

In the controlled environment of the Sleep Disorders Center, Schenck and his colleagues watch patients gorge on chips and soda. But when sleep eaters are at home, says Schenck, the menu gets really bizarre: cat food sandwiches, sometimes salted, and the eggshell and coffee ground smoothies we mentioned above. Non-food items can also tempt the sleep eater— sometimes dangerously so. Schenck has had patients eat Elmer's Glue, a bar of soap, and medications. "Inedible substances are consumed, because they look appetizing to the person without a proper judgment," he says.

Doctors classify sleep eating as a *sleep* disorder, not an eating disorder, although researchers are puzzling over a possible link between the daytime eating disorders (bulimia nervosa and anorexia) and sleep eating. All these disorders are much more common in women (70 percent of sleep eaters are female). Why? So far, science is baffled.

The fact that sleep eaters gravitate toward junk food or comfort food is unfortunate. The sleep eater quickly puts on weight. "These people love thick foods," says Schenck. "Peanut butter, whole milk, milk shakes, pies, pasta. All the kinds of comfort foods are preferentially consumed in sleep eating. Fruits and vegetables are thrown on the floor with disdain."

Over all the years of binging on fatty foods, Amy has not gained any excess weight. She is the lucky exception, not the rule. Most sleep eaters struggle with both their weight and body image.

ANNA RYAN

Anna Ryan, who works in a family landscaping business with her husband Kenny in Missouri, has put on sixty pounds in the last year and a half. She now has high blood pressure and is a prime candidate for diabetes. Plus, she's exhausted.

At first, Anna didn't even know that she was sleep eating. "I'd wake up and it felt like I hadn't gone to bed," she says. "By noon, I just was exhausted. I work in a family business, and I'd tell my dad: 'I'm going home.' And everybody kept saying, 'What's wrong with you?'"

Unaware of how many times she was getting up each night, Anna was brave enough (and curious enough!) to let us put night vision cameras into her home to find out. What we saw was astonishing. At 2 A.M., Anna got out of her bed, fast asleep. She headed straight to the kitchen—one of five hungry prowls we recorded over a two-night period.

During a typical night, her husband, Kenny, a heavy sleeper (a "tornado" wouldn't wake him up, Anna says), doesn't notice that Anna is up and about. Like most sleep eaters, she gravitates toward the high-calorie foods. When we filmed her, she had a yen for snack bars, which she ate with abandon, never waking up. She even took them to bed.

"What does it feel like when you wake up in the morning and you see the wrappers and realize what you've done?" we asked her.

"Upset," she replied. "It's upsetting. And I get frustrated with myself. You feel like you should be able to control it."

Of course, Anna hadn't seen herself sleep-eat until we showed her the tape. The images shocked her.

"How embarrassing," she said. "I wonder why I don't choke. I didn't realize I was in bed eating and then laying down, eating. It's a little scarier than I thought, actually."

Anna and Kenny have stopped buying junk food, but it doesn't matter. Anna sleep eats anything: cereals, frozen foods, whatever is on hand. "We've put locks on certain cabinets that have high-caloric foods, but you can't put locks on every single cabinet in your kitchen, and your refrigerator and freezer," Anna says.

She's tried altering her eating habits to ward off her sleep eating. "Being in the lawn and garden business, you work long hours, and then in the evening tend to eat a bigger meal.

I still get up in the middle of the night. It doesn't matter what I eat. I've tried eating nothing all day long. That way I could just live off my calories at night. And that doesn't work. I tried eating big meals through the day and being really full, hoping that maybe my brain would say *you're full* and I wouldn't get up. And I still get up."

TREATMENTS

The biggest barrier to treating SRED is getting a diagnosis—is it just sleep eating, or is it also sleepwalking, restless leg syndrome, or sleep apnea? Is the sleep eater taking any medication that is causing her to prowl the kitchen in the night? In some instances, sleeping pills have been shown to lead to the kind of blended states of waking and sleep that can induce SRED.

"You want to identify what we call co-morbidity," says Schenck, "any associated condition, and correct it. Often, that will control the associated sleep eating. There's also a medication—an antiseizure and migraine medicine called Topamax—topiramate is [the] generic name—that has a very, very strong property in controlling abnormal eating during the day and at night."

Schenck began treating Amy, the teacher we introduced you to above, with a dopamine medication to control her restless leg syndrome (which, by the way, she shares with her father), but it did not control her sleep eating. Schenck says that Amy's SRED was so ingrained that she needed topiramate to control her sleep eating.

"It has worked wonders," Amy says. "It's something that I'm definitely not gonna be cured from where I could stop taking pills. It's something that you definitely are just going to have to learn to live with. Some days I wonder why. Other days I think God has given me the restless legs and sleep eating to spread the word."

. . . the word that you're not sentenced to a lifetime of eating frozen egg rolls and ketchup in a trance at 3 A.M.

As for Anna, it took months, but doctors found a medication that seems to work for her. She says she's sleeping through the night and the pounds are coming off. She has two bags of her "before" clothes that she is hanging on to. "Once they get a grip on this, I'm going back to my old weight," Anna says. "I never was skin and bones. I mean, I'm a robust Italian woman," she laughs. "I will get back to my old clothes. I guarantee it."

That day may be fast approaching. Anna's kitchen is calm, quiet, and undisturbed all night long.

21. TRICHOTILLOMANIA

WE ALL OCCASIONALLY TOUCH, FIDDLE WITH, TWIRL, OR TUG ON a lock of our hair. A harmless habit, for most of us—but it's a draining, debilitating medical condition for those with an unlucky neurological condition. They don't just tug or twirl—they pull out their hair, even their eyelashes. They can't stop, and have no idea why—a medical mystery with the unpronounceable name of trichotillomania, "trich" for short.

I first came across this strange affliction years ago—in a "Dear Abby" column. As you can imagine, it stuck in my mind—and we remembered that another ABC show had covered the topic. It gave us the perfect opportunity to reexamine the affliction and do a follow-up on a fascinating woman who had used the first TV report to turn her life around.

Trich is not quite as rare as you might think. Estimates say it afflicts 1 to 3 percent of Americans, mostly women. People who have it often take refuge in wigs or hats, so you may know a trich sufferer and not even be aware of it. It's *not* a psychological problem or a "bad habit": it's medical—a neurological disorder in the same family as obsessive-compulsive disorder (OCD) or Tourette's syndrome (which produces repetitive, involuntary movements or verbal outbursts called tics that may have genetic roots).

People with trich literally can't help themselves—despite their best (and most creative) efforts, their hands inexorably move to their heads and pluck individual hairs out by their roots, over and over and over. To show that the chic and beautiful are not exempt, we asked a beauty queen and Hollywood stylist to share their stories. They were, amazingly, happy to: they wanted people living with trich in shame and silence to know that they're not alone.

MANDI LINE

Mandi Line is the woman who had talked to ABC about trichotillomania years ago. She was always pretty and popular, a child model, homecoming queen, beauty pageant winner, and successful Hollywood stylist. She had a funky, eclectic look—cool clothes, hot pink sections of hair, stylish hats. She made stars look good by day—and at night, in the privacy of her home, she felt compelled to secretly pull out her own hair, even eyebrows.

In that long-ago interview with our correspondent Juju Chang, Mandi had "outed" herself on national television, removing her hat and fake hairpieces to show that entire areas of her head were completely bald and other areas had hair barely a quarter inch long. Taking off a wig or hat in front of someone else is one of the hardest things a person with trich can do. Twenty-eight years old at the time of that first interview, Mandi had only shown her bare head to her mother and an ex-boyfriend. Weeping and taking a deep breath, Mandi got ready to take off her "disguise."

"Tell me why you're crying," Juju said to her.

"Because you're sitting here interviewing this girl and you think she's one person," she replied. "And then, all of a sudden, I'm going to be someone else."

"Who will you become?"

"Me. But what I think is the ugly version of me. Oh God, just do it." And the hat came off. Then the hair, artfully arranged to hide the bald spots, was swept aside. All that was left was her hot pink clip-ons in the front, and Mandi decided to go for a complete revelation.

"Screw it. There are my little bangs."

Off the clips came. Chang gently asked Mandi what it felt like, revealing herself in this way.

"It's like I'm naked," said Mandi. "This is all my damage from last night." One half of her head had been covered with "peach fuzz," hair that was growing in. Mandi had pulled it all out.

When we showed Mandi this tape of herself, from years before, she felt almost like it was an interview with another person. "It's so funny," she said. "I was thinking how long ago this was. That girl back then cried. It's so heartbreaking when I see it. [I] was so scared of what people would think after that interview. [Now] I can say I'm a different person."

The difference between the first and second interviews? Mandi has accepted herself in ways that would have been inconceivable before she "went public." She has become a role model for people with trich, who come up to her on the street, grab her hand, and thank her for destigmatizing the disorder.

A PHYSICAL SYNDROME

When she was young, doctors told Mandi that her trich was a psychological problem. Doctors had absolutely no idea what the disorder was about, and she remembers being offered some strange theories: "I had a therapist tell me when I was seven that I wasn't sexually comfortable with myself yet. I was seven years old. What did I even know?"

Trich seems to start innocently enough. Mandi remembers her first moments with it: watching *The Greatest American Hero* as a child and casually pulling on her hair.

Dr. Nancy Keuthen is the codirector of the Trichotillomania Clinic at Mass General and an associate professor of psychology in the Department of Psychiatry at Harvard Medical School. She says the causes of the disorder and why it has onset at a particular time, in a particular setting, for one person and not another, are puzzles that researchers are trying to solve.

"Trichotillomania is such a medical mystery because we still know very little about the genetics and the biology of it," Keuthen says. "It's a physical syndrome inside the brain. Not psychiatric."

Keuthen gives us the clinical definition of the disorder: "It's characterized by repetitive hair pulling that results in noticeable hair loss. Generally, the sufferer says that they have urges prior to pulling or when attempting to resist the impulse. They experience pleasure, relief, or gratification upon pulling."

While her typical patient is female with the onset in early adolescence, Keuthen has seen babies with the disorder, and she's seen its onset in octogenarians.

Why is trich more common in females? We place such a great importance on girls and hair: is that why this syndrome is expressed this way in this gender? Or is it influenced by hormonal differences between the two sexes? Keuthen suspects the gender issue may be inflated and men may have just as much trich as women. After all, men can conceal their hair loss. "They can attribute it to male pattern baldness," she says. "That is much more difficult for girls and women." In addition, the records on which the statistics are based tend to be clinical, from hospitals and doctors' offices. That may skew the sample all on its own; women are more likely than men to seek treatment, so doctors will see higher numbers for trich in women.

A GROOMING GENE GONE AWRY?

There is a theory that trich is caused by a "grooming" gene that we all carry that has somehow gone awry. We don't necessarily think of ourselves as grooming in the way animals do. But you don't have to look further than the multibillion-dollar cosmetics industry or the astronomical sums we spend on hair care to realize we may not be as far from chimpanzees picking lice off each other as we like to imagine.

Keuthen notes analogies to trich in the animal kingdom. "There's canine acral lick," says Keuthen. "There's feline alopecia. There's avian feather picking. Mice may pluck the fur of cage mates. Or, if they're housed singly, they'll pluck their own fur."

To try to understand this behavior, researchers have worked with animals. They've tried eliminating the function of a gene named Hox-B8 in mice. That change causes "barbering behavior" that is similar to trich in humans. Hox-B8 may be one of many genes involved in the disorder.

That made us wonder: what purpose does grooming serve? The removal of parasites, of course. But grooming may also serve complex social functions that have to do with the cohesion of the group and the establishment of different kinds of bonds, including sexual bonds, between individuals.

"There's an evolutionary basis to grooming," says Keuthen. "But in the humans that have trichotillomania, it's gone awry, and it's excessive, and there's no functional basis to it."

TRIGGERS

Why do trich patients pull?

Some of Keuthen's patients say it's a way of reducing stress. Others experience gratification or pleasure from pulling. Mandi mentioned boredom as a trigger.

Keuthen says the impulse to pull is very difficult to control: "People say that they experience pleasure or relief when they do it. It's cheap. It's under their control."

The most common place to pull is the hair behind the ears. Keuthen has seen an almost addictive attachment to a certain place on the scalp. Her patients return to it again and again, and it becomes sensitized. It's a cruel irony that trich sufferers often experience guilt when they're pulling, and that very guilt drives them to pull even more. When the hair regrows, it is often with a different texture or color, which may also provoke the behavior.

JENA METTS

If you saw Jena Metts, a student from Kentucky, you'd probably envy her. She's bubbly, blond, poised, great-looking. But she has the same secret as other trich patients. She pulls out her own hair. A resourceful person, she has tried every trick you can think of to keep her pulling under control, from wearing gloves to taping her fingers together. (Mandi told us, by the way, that she actually has calluses on her fingers from pulling her hair.) Jena wears a tight, knitted beanie hat at night to try to disrupt her compulsion.

"Whenever I get emotional, very stressed, or upset—I go for my hair," says Jena. "And sometimes if there's like a little hair sticking up, I want to pull it. Whenever I'm super bored at home, I pull."

It changed Jena's life when she saw the 2003 ABC piece on Mandi. Jena reached out through ABC's offices, and Mandi responded. Jena had harbored a dream of being a beauty queen, but she had been afraid to pursue it because of her trich. With Mandi's example and encouragement, she took a deep breath and entered the Miss Kentucky pageant. We watched her compete—blocking the big dance number, mingling with the other contestants, grinning.

Mandi has this to say about her protégé: "Jena's gonna be ten times the lady I am. Jena is skyrocketing."

Jena says the pageant was a watershed for her. At first it was hard to tell her fellow contestants about her condition. But she remembered that she wanted to be open about it— and though contest rules said she *could* wear a wig, she decided not to. She wanted her presence to say, in a very public way: this is who I am, and I'm not ashamed of it. "Once I said it, and it was kind of out there, it felt like water under the bridge," says Jena.

One of the reasons she competed was because trich is such a disfiguring disorder. "A lot of people who have it are ashamed of it," she says. "They feel like they can't live a normal life."

Jena didn't get the crown, but she still feels like she won something.

"To be honest, the whole experience has been really uplifting," she says. "And if I had a chance, I'd do it again."

SUPPORT GROUPS

There are trich support groups across the county. We visited one in Los Angeles called HEART (Helping Educate And Reach out to Trichsters) where we met member Rosalina Castillo, who has an odd variation of trich, pulling out her eyelashes, as well as its more common form of pulling hair from the scalp. Rosalina has worn wigs to hide her bald spots, but she went through high school afraid of being discovered. As a teenager, she was teased: "I would have comments like 'Are you wearing a wig?' 'I think she's wearing a wig. We should find out. Maybe we should pull her wig off and see.'" Rosalina says she doesn't date because she's scared of rejection.

The support group helps its members cope, giving them activities such as sign language and jewelry-making to keep their hands busy. It can also be a safe setting to take that first step toward self-acceptance.

Rosalina showed us what she looked like without her wig. Her lively face, surrounded by clouds of dark, wavy hair, was just as beautiful when the hairpiece was taken off—and you could be forgiven if you thought her super-short hair was a daring haircut. But it's taken her *years* to feel comfortable without artificial hair—to feel like she could show us the "real" Rosalina.

APRIL DARLING was another member of HEART, only thirteen years old when we interviewed her. She says she pulls her hair mostly from behind her ears. Her disorder baffles her. "How could I stop?" she asks. "What was making me do this? There was a demon inside of me saying: 'Pull out your hair!'"

Her mother tried to help her by giving her little toys to play with to keep her hands busy. The toys would sometimes work, but usually the little voice in her head would tell her: "You've got to pull. It will make you feel better."

April often wonders: why me? But she sees an upside: she does say that grappling with the "little demon" has made her a better person. "I think it's made me a lot stronger," she says. "More caring. More loving."

IS THERE A CURE?

A cure is not something trich sufferers count on. Some interventions—such as antidepressant/antianxiety medications (selective serotonin reuptake inhibitors) or cognitive behavior therapy can be effective in helping some people sporadically manage the behavior.

"Honestly, I think our treatments right now are somewhat underwhelming in their efficacy," says Dr. Keuthen. "We're really in our infancy in developing treatments. Our treatments can help in the short run. But most of the research shows that the benefits don't endure."

Medications used for obsessive-compulsive disorder and Tourette's are sometimes effective. These medicines balance certain chemicals in the brain. But behavior treatments are just as important. There are generally two types—"habit reversal" or "habit control training." Therapists try to heighten patients' awareness of what they are doing and when they are doing it. When are they likely to pull? When does the urge come? When are they manipulating their hair? Therapists then try to replace the trich hand activity— pulling—with something else *incompatible* with pulling hair: making a fist, for example. Therapists also try to find a support network for what can be a very long process of breaking stubbornly habituated behaviors.

There are also therapies called stimulus control techniques, which involve spending as much time as possible in public settings where the urge to pull is inhibited by the awareness that people are watching. Activities where the hands are free—such as watching TV—are discouraged.

Trich sufferers wear hats that cover the places from which they're likely to pull. They also wear gloves or bandages on their hands in an effort to keep themselves from pulling. And, of course, trich tends to strike when people are anxious, upset, or frustrated. People have suggested that it may be a

way of managing those emotions. So it can help to keep sufferers on an emotionally even keel.

The bad news is that it doesn't go away, although in some
cases with children it can be what researchers call "self-
limiting" and their trich will disappear over time. In adults,
once it starts, that's it—you've got it for life.

We saw in Mandi and Jena that one of the most important
things trich sufferers can learn is self-acceptance. HEART
has helped Rosalina and April learn that hard lesson, too. "I
used to care so much what other people would think of me,"
April says. "Now I just think—everybody has their opinion
and they can think whatever they want. I'm not changing for
them."

As for the hair pulling of our original patient, Mandi, still
glamorous and chic, she says she now has bad weeks and good
weeks. At one point, she improved so much that she considered giving modeling another try. Then the trich came back.

Is there a cure out there for her? "I don't want people to
give up hope," she says. "There are some people who have
stopped. But I don't think I'm going to stop. I just think that
I need to be a better me. But cured? I don't know."

22. TOO MUCH NOISE

ACUTE SENSES ARE TERRIFIC THINGS—PEOPLE TAKE PRIDE IN keen vision or a refined sense of taste. A musician might take great delight in a heightened sense of hearing.

But what if you could hear things nobody else could hear—things you didn't *want* to hear? What if you could hear everything that was happening inside your body? If your own heart's every beat sounded deep inside you? If every step you took reverberated inside your head? If every breath drowned out your wife's words, and you could hear your own eyes moving in their sockets?

That's what happened to musician Adrian McLeish, an Englishman who plays first French horn in an orchestra in Kassel, Germany. Adrian remembers the very moment these bizarre sound effects began. It was twenty-three years ago, five years after he had joined the Kassel orchestra.

"I was practicing my horn one day," says Adrian, "and I had this strange sensation that I was hearing my horn playing somehow on the *inside* of my head."

The music was distorted; his own voice began echoing like a kazoo, with an unpleasant buzzing vibration that he felt inside his skull.

It got more and more extreme. Imagine his world: when he combed his hair, he could hear the scratching of the comb against his scalp, as though he were listening from *inside* his body. When he ate something crunchy, it sounded like a gunshot through his brain. But the oddest sound happened one night as he was reading.

"I thought we had a mouse in the wall," says Adrian. "Every few seconds I heard a scratching noise. Every time I stopped to listen, the scratching stopped. Then, I realized what was happening. I could hear my eyeballs moving in their sockets!"

A MUSICIAN'S NIGHTMARE

Adrian's own voice became like a cracked loudspeaker inside the left side of his head. It didn't vary in pitch or volume, so he couldn't hear what his voice sounded like to others. The sound of his own chewing made it difficult to converse during meals. His French horn's lovely timbre was amplified and sounded like a buzz saw. It was pure torture going to the dentist to have his teeth polished.

He had to give up jogging: the combination of his footfalls registering deafeningly, his heart pounding, and the sound of his lungs rasping inside his head was too much to bear.

In addition to all the auditory problems assaulting him, Adrian also had what's called Tullio's phenomenon: his visual world moved in sync with the distorted clamor in his head. Every sound he heard inside his body made his eyes jump around.

"My eyes were jerking with my speech," he says. "If I played a series of notes on the horn, my eyes would jump up and down."

That problem prevented Adrian from doing his job—he couldn't read music anymore.

"If somebody sat next to me and played drum or a trombone or stood behind me and sang, the notes in front of me would jump up and down in time with what I was hearing," says Adrian. "So if I had to play something fast, or someone next to me was playing something loud, I couldn't read the music. I had to play fast things from memory. I was once doing a choral concert. The choir was standing right behind the orchestra. A soprano singing right behind me had a particular vibrato. My part was jumping up and down, waving in time with her music. It was accompanied by the feeling of a needle being stuck in [my] ear. The combination [was] awful—it was never just one thing."

Still, music was Adrian's life, and his profession. He continued to play through the discomfort and pain.

SHOTS IN THE DARK

Adrian's case stumped doctor after doctor. One gave him tranquilizers. Another suggested he drink more beer. In desperation, Adrian even tried a faith healer, who told him that he was a victim of sorcery and that there was a demon working like a parasite inside his head, which a colleague had planted there to sabotage him in his job (and that will be $100, please).

It was the jumping in his eyes that finally convinced his doctors that Adrian's problem was serious. He endured three operations—unfortunately, all were for the wrong diagnosis.

"They tried to patch me up," says Adrian. "And it was well meant, but in the wrong place."

Doctors in Munich opened up his eardrum looking for a fistula, a leak between middle and inner ear which could have been responsible for the eye movements Adrian was experiencing. They didn't find a leak, but they tried to stabilize Adrian's hearing mechanism. Something called a stirrup— one of three tiny bones in your ear that moves to transform the vibrations of sound into the electrical signals your brain can interpret—had come loose. The surgeons patched it with pieces of cartilage and glue.

"This dampened my hearing and these phenomena minutely, for a very short time," says Adrian. "The second operation a year later helped the same amount of time, just a few weeks."

It was during the third operation that a surgeon put a piece of silicon foam in Adrian's ear, which, he says, allowed him to continue working. "I was partially deaf in one ear," he says. "I was immune to loud sounds from the outside. Things I played myself didn't disturb me quite as much. But it didn't help the autophony: I still heard myself very, very loudly."

Adrian thinks that is what finally caused his tinnitus, a static buzzing or scratching sound, which started in 1995 and got worse and worse, until Adrian had to quit the orchestra and put down his beloved horn.

"I finally had to capitulate," Adrian says. "I threw in the towel. The day had come when I just couldn't carry on."

THE MIRACLE OF THE WEB

It was on a particularly bad day that Adrian went looking on the Web for someone else in the world with his set of symptoms.

"I typed in autophony, Tullio, and tinnitus," says Adrian—three words his doctors had made him all too familiar with. "This is no exaggeration, within twenty-five seconds, I knew I'd found it. All my symptoms were described. I remember saying it out loud, 'I found it.' After twenty-two years, this had to be it."

The "it" that Adrian had found was superior canal dehiscence, SCD, a defect in the bone of the inner ear. It was a syndrome that hadn't even been named when Adrian began having symptoms. Dr. Lloyd Minor of Johns Hopkins Medical Center in Baltimore had discovered and named the syndrome in the 1990s, so Adrian immediately made plans to go there for treatment.

"I thought, it's a perfect testament to how patients are helping us so much in making diagnoses," Minor comments. "Mr. McLeish found us by simply going to Google and typing in keywords. He came up with our work and superior canal dehiscence and contacted me. Getting medical information out today is so much different than it was even as recently as five or ten years ago."

If you look through the chapters of this book, you'll see that's remarkably true. Patients who are suffering from a bizarre set of symptoms can often find out what ails them with a few clicks. Of course, there's a related syndrome: cyberchondria. You know you have it when you constantly enter your symptoms into Internet sites and decide that your aches, fever, and runny nose are dengue fever.

THE INNER GYROSCOPE

Most of us take our ears and hearing for granted. We think sound waves go into our ear canals, vibrate our eardrums, the vibrations are changed into electrical signals, and we hear—the same way our music systems work. But the complicated system of ear canals and bones was here long before your MP3 player; it's a lot more complex, and it does more than hear.

Each of our ears contains three fluid-filled canals that sense our position in three-dimensional space. That's what keeps us balanced when we move, without our ever thinking about it. "They're like a gyroscope in an airplane," says Minor. "And every time we move our head, even by a minute amount, these receptors tell the brain exactly how the head is moving."

In Adrian's case, Minor determined, the gyroscope was damaged—a leak existed between canals. A sliver of bone was missing in his left superior canal, so the fluid, separated only by a thin membrane, was actually touching Adrian's brain. Instead of being insulated by bone, every sound was going through the fluid in the superior canal and being transmitted, physically, right to his brain.

"The ear canal, when there's an opening in it, can act like an amplifier for sound," Minor says. Voilà: buzzing voice, thumping heartbeat, scratchy eye sounds.

"The ear canals are at roughly right angles to one another," Minor explains. The top "balance canal" is called the superior semicircle canal ("superior" because it's in the upper portion of the ear), and patients with SCD have an absence of bone covering that top balance canal. Ordinarily, this canal only senses angular motion of the head: where you are in space. When there's an opening in the bone, though, the canal can respond to sound vibrations and pressure, and act like an amplifier.

Not much is supposed to move inside your ear; normal ears have only two spots with mobility. One is a structure called the "oval window," which is where that stirrup bone attaches to the inner ear. The other is called the "round window." Sound goes in through the oval window, around through the cochlea, the hearing organ, and out through the round window. But patients with SCD have a third mobile window—that hole in the superior semicircular canal. So sound can get in through the stirrup bone/oval window *and* through the dehiscence, the opening in the bone.

And why did Adrian's eyes move every time he heard something? The minute pulses in the fluid of Adrian's brain caused tiny movements of the fluid in the balance canal. Movement in the balance canal sends us the message "Hey, my body is moving." The eyes were moving to help figure out where the body was in space.

Think of the canal as a tire, with an inner tube and a hard outer layer. The hard outer layer is the bone that covers the canal—inside it's liquid. In patients with SCD, part of the outer layer is missing and the inner layer is in direct contact with the lining of the brain.

SCD seems to be a problem that develops over time. Roughly three quarters of the patients Minor sees have it in only one ear; the rest have it in both ears. Minor has found that even when his patients have the syndrome in only one ear, the bone covering the other balance canal is abnormally thin. When you look at a broad spectrum of patients, you see that it isn't as rare as you might imagine: about a thousand *autopsy* reports in general patients reported that bone thinness when they went looking for it. Minor notes, however, that the syndrome is very rare in children.

"Either it's not being picked up, or, more likely, it just doesn't exist in children," he says. "So perhaps there's a thin layer of bone that over the course of time, say from the pressure of the brain, or from things that cause pulsations of the brain, may become eroded or disrupted. When that happens, then we get the full manifestation of dehiscence."

The typical age of onset is forty. For Adrian, his symptoms began when he was a bit younger. He'd been living with SCD for much of his adult life. But, finally, diagnosis in hand, Adrian and his wife planned a trip to Baltimore to see Minor.

SURGERY

Adrian was probably born with a predilection for SCD—the bone in his ear canal was just too thin. As he aged, the bone wore down and a hole developed. The solution to the problem? Surgery.

At Hopkins, Minor has seen 145 patients with the syndrome, and he's operated on 48 of those. Whether or not to operate depends on the patient: Is the patient debilitated by the symptoms of SCD? Is he no longer able to carry out activities that are important to his life? That's the time to consider surgery. If it's a mild nuisance, if the patient can control it by simply putting an earplug in when going to a concert or a football game, then there's probably no need to operate.

Adrian felt the operation was his last chance at saving his career. Sound was, after all, his livelihood. But beyond that, he hoped that the operation could finally quiet the daily chaos inside his head.

Minor had been the one to originally identify and describe the syndrome, so one look at the scans of Adrian's head showed him that his was a pretty clear-cut case. Minor was able to point to an indentation in the bone—the tiny defect that had caused Adrian so much grief.

"This little trench right here, is the dehiscence," says Minor. "We actually plug the canal, and we do that analogous to the way you would fix a pothole in the road."

This "pothole" surgery is fairly straightforward, although there is the risk of hearing loss. "One classic teaching in otology and neurotology is that you're trying *not* to get into the inner ear when you can avoid it," says Minor. "Yet nature has already opened the inner ear in these patients. So just working in that area carries some risk of hearing loss. Another complication is bleeding. This is an area in which even a small accumulation of blood has to be dealt with quickly and evacuated in order to make sure that the patient doesn't have any swelling, infection. And finally, since we are working around the brain, stroke or seizure or memory disturbance or language disturbance are always potential complications. But by being able to navigate very accurately in the operation, the amount of retraction on the brain (that is, the amount they need to 'move' the brain tissue) is minimal during these surgeries."

His wife seemed nervous, but Adrian was his usual self just before the surgery—he even joked, "Will I ever play the piano again?" Which, for a French horn player about to undergo surgery near his brain, we thought was pretty funny.

The operation went off without a hitch, the doctors filling the hole with some of Adrian's own tissue and some man-made material. But Adrian would have to wait to see if it would work. With so many bandages around his head and ear, it was hard to tell right away if the surgery had been successful. A lot depended on what Adrian would hear—and would *not* hear—in the days after the recovery room.

A NEW MAN

A week after his surgery, Adrian is amazed. "It is a miracle," he says. "The noises are gone. I do not hear my voice. I do not hear my heartbeat. I don't hear chewing. I don't hear my footsteps when I walk. All those things I heard for twenty-three years in my left ear have gone."

Finally, he can hear the welcome sound of silence.

Minor confirms that Adrian's ear is now repaired. And his eyes? Finally steady.

We watch as Adrian pours out his gratitude to Minor.

"I thank you from the bottom of my heart," Adrian says. "I can start jogging again. I can't hear my eyes move anymore. That's gone. And now I'm looking forward to getting back to my playing. There's an orchestra waiting for me."

Adrian got a hero's welcome, when, eight months after his surgery, he returned to his first French horn seat in Kassel. Finally, he hears the music—and only the music.

It was a long road for Adrian, but he feels reborn.

"I got my life back," he says.

And we all got to think about how grateful we are that we *don't* know every single thing that our bodies are doing for us every moment. I'm delighted that my eyes can move around, but, thank you, I don't need to hear it!

23. FATAL FAMILIAL INSOMNIA

D O YOU REMEMBER THE LAST TIME YOU HAD A COMPLETELY SLEEPLESS night and how bad you felt the next day? Try to imagine not sleeping for months.

We've covered a number of medical mysteries that focus on sleep disorders, but fatal familial insomnia is perhaps the most disturbing of them. It could have been dreamed up by Edgar Allan Poe—a Gothic nightmare that affects only forty families around the world, all of whom have a mutant gene that has been passed down through the generations. It causes those who inherit it to endure a fatal form of insomnia—yes, *fatal*.

Like a poison fruit, the genetic mutation for FFI hangs on their family tree. The odds of inheriting it are fifty-fifty. If you do inherit it, when will it strike? What triggers it? Doctors don't know. They do know that once the disease takes hold it's impossible to stop it. It tears through the brain, impairing the ability to move, talk, and sleep, and eventually kills its victims.

THE SISTERS

Cheryl and Carolyn are adult sisters—they asked us not to divulge their last name. They have lived for years with the disease hanging over them. They didn't know about it when they were young, but in 1999, it tragically revealed itself in their mother, Barbara.

Inside Barbara's brain, a genetic trip wire had been crossed. In a matter of months, she went from being a vigorous fifty-two-year-old woman to being completely incapacitated, in a coma from which she emerged for only a few days, right before she died.

Cheryl recalls those last days in the hospital: "They took her intubation out. She couldn't really talk because she was so dry-throated. And she wrote: 'FFI?'"

Neither sister knew about the condition, but they soon found out that it had killed their grandfather and their uncle. Barbara, their mother, didn't know when she died if she had passed along the disease to either daughter, or both. She also didn't know that each would have the chance to find out if the fatal gene was in every strand of DNA in her body.

PATIENT ZERO

To understand this disease, we should start in Italy, two hundred fifty years ago. Researchers believe a wealthy Venetian doctor, whose name has been kept secret, unknowingly carried the original genetic mutation for FFI. Experts simply refer to him as "Patient Zero," the first known case of the disease. By the time he died in 1765, he had passed the gene, and the curse, to his children. The chain had begun.

In its first stages, stricken family members experienced a recognizable kind of insomnia. But common sleeplessness quickly became something completely uncommon—an endless parade of nights and days without any sleep at all.

"I'd say within a month, it's pretty clear that you've got a disease like no other," says D. T. Max, an author in Washington, DC, who has spent years researching FFI. His book, *The Family That Couldn't Sleep*, traces the Italian clan who first carried the disease—and is a fascinating meditation on sleep, fate, and mortality.

"One, you're not sleeping," says Max. "Two, you're having difficulty walking. Three, your ability to focus has gone downhill rapidly. Ordinarily, in the ninth month, the disease ends in death."

We first heard of FFI in a magazine article Daniel Max wrote when he was researching the book. That article first brought our attention to the fact that insomnia can kill you. Max had fascinating details to share.

Many of the afflicted Italian family members were brought to San Servolo, an island asylum a short boat ride from Venice. Now a museum, San Servolo feels almost haunted.

Max came with us to Venice, and mused about what it must have been like to walk inside San Servolo's walls.

"There would be howls," he says. "There would be people doing unintended behavior. There would be attendants chasing after them."

In one room downstairs there were leather restraints on a bed. FFI patients, as the condition moves forward, are often not quite fully asleep but not really awake either. They can wander around in a daze unless something holds them down.

"Generation after generation in this family in the later stages of the disease were strapped to a bed at night," says Max.

Records show that throughout the eighteenth, nineteenth, and twentieth centuries, deaths consistent with FFI ran down through the generations of this unlucky Venetian family. Then, in the 1980s, a descendant, whose first name was Silvano, learned that he was affected, too. This handsome, vibrant playboy had lived in the shadow of this potential killer all his life.

Max brought us to Dr. Elio Lugaresi, director of the Neurology Clinic at the University of Bologna. He shared some remarkable footage: a film of Silvano, in the throes of the disease. They had filmed him, and other members of the family, at the University of Bologna's Sleep Clinic.

Lugaresi spoke to us through a translator. "Silvano looks as if he's sleepwalking," Lugaresi says. "That's really because he's in a permanent state of pre-sleep behavior. Often, you will see him and other patients performing gestures like combing their hair or washing their hands or handling objects." We watched, fascinated, as Silvano, eyes half-open, seemed to mime buttoning his shirt, brushing his hair.

FFI's victims have a desperate problem: they are unable to drop into a deep REM sleep. What about sleeping pills? In a cruel irony, sleep medications only accelerate their restless descent toward death. When Lugaresi gave these patients intravenous doses of barbiturates to try to help them sleep, they went into a deep coma without ever passing through the revitalizing REM stage of sleep they so desperately needed.

Victims of FFI are forever trying and failing to fall asleep. Before dying, they hover for months in a twilight world. But just before his death, Silvano made an offer that would change the course of the disease for all FFI sufferers. He asked researchers to study his brain after he died. It finally opened a window into the mystery of a centuries-old specter.

DEADLY PRIONS

With Silvano's brain and those of other sufferers, scientists could finally try to isolate the problem. Their conclusion? A tiny geometric difference in a protein.

Healthy proteins, like all large molecules, have a shape— long or twisted or folded or smooth. But one protein, triggered by genetic mutations, "mis-folds." It becomes the wrong shape, which, it turns out, affects its function, creating what doctors call an abnormal prion. Prions can replicate themselves, and these abnormal proteins infect the brain and form clumps. They destroy nerve cells and eventually leave sponge-like holes in the brain. You may have heard of some other prion diseases: mad cow, Creutzfeldt-Jakob disease, and kuru.

Dr. Michael Geschwind, a neurologist at the Memory and Aging Center at the University of California San Francisco Medical Center, studies FFI. He explains prions and what they do.

"A prion is a protein that sits on the surface of a cell," says Geschwind. "It's on most cells of the body. The brain, in particular, has a very high number of prion proteins."

Usually when doctors talk about prions, they're talking about the aberrant ones, the abnormally shaped prions that cause disease. Geschwind says the function of prions is still not completely known. "Scientists in the laboratory can actually remove the gene that encodes the prion protein, so that a mouse will develop without any prion protein," he says. "And those mice were initially thought to be completely normal."

It turned out, however, that the mice did have some deficits and abnormalities. The normal prion protein probably plays some role in memory and in learning. And it also likely plays a role in protecting a cell from stress or injury. For example, experiments have shown that animals without prion proteins have much more severe damage from a stroke.

Scientists have known about the diseases abnormal prions can cause since the early 1900s. "We knew about [the] diseases," says Geschwind, "but we didn't know that they were caused by a misshapen protein. It was work by Stanley Prusiner here at UCSF and others around the world that helped determine that these diseases, which used to be called 'transmissible spongiform encephalopathies,' or TSEs, were actually caused by a misshapen protein."

For years, researchers thought the diseases were caused by slow viruses. "Prusiner and others," says Geschwind, "demonstrated that you could actually treat material from these patients in a way that would kill viruses [and] bacteria." But when researchers took a piece of treated brain tissue from a patient who had died from the disease and injected it into an animal, it contracted the disease. That meant the disease wasn't caused by a virus or bacteria. "Only when you treated the material in a way that changed the shape of proteins (what

we call 'denatured proteins') could you actually prevent trans-
mission of the disease," says Geschwind.

Geschwind says that he's trying to find ways of diagnosing
the disease early on. "One of my goals is to try to identify the
very earliest features of the disease—maybe even features
that occur before a patient or a family member is aware that
they are occurring. In a patient who carries a mutation, but is
not yet symptomatic, maybe there are some early markers that
are occurring, such as an increase in certain proteins in the
blood. Maybe [there are] changes on MRI or other imaging of
the brain. And maybe that would be the time to start treatment."

When we interviewed Geschwind, he and his lab were
embarked on clinical trials for a drug called quinicrine, one
of the medicines that Prusiner's laboratory discovered which
has been shown to be effective at removing prions from cells.
"We have started the first ever treatment trial for prion disease in the United States," says Geschwind, adding that research into FFI and prion diseases may eventually lead to
breakthroughs in more common disorders, like Alzheimer's
and Parkinson's.

A TOUGH CHOICE

Most of the damage from misfolded prions in FFI seems to
be in an area of the brain called the thalamus. The thalamus,
not surprisingly, is the region of the brain responsible for the
regulation of sleep—why Silvano's family's and Barbara's
sleep function went haywire.

The sisters were confronted with a thorny choice: a blood test can now reveal early markers that will tell whether or not they carry the FFI gene. When Max first began interviewing them years ago, neither sister knew if she had inherited that gene from their mother. (For reasons not fully understood, symptoms of FFI don't show up until midlife, after child-bearing years: it hadn't, as yet, become active in Barbara's daughters.)

Ask yourself: would you want to know if you have the FFI gene? Each sister made a different choice.

Carolyn, pregnant with her second child, decided for the sake of the kids, and to be able to plan for her future, to test to see if she carried the gene. Cheryl didn't want to know.

"I do or do not have this disease," says Cheryl. "It cannot define me. If it's my story, I get to choose whether I laugh or cry about it. It's my choice. I'm going to laugh about it. It's my day. It's my life. I can die in a car accident on the way home. I may just as easily die from cancer. We all have a terminal something. That's the way it goes."

Cheryl, who is younger than Carolyn, says their different decisions "wreaked havoc" on their relationship.

We interviewed the sisters together. As you can imagine, the decision was a burden to both, and each initially questioned the other sister's choice.

"When I first found out that you wanted to know, I was furious," Cheryl admits. "I thought it was hellacious. How could I tell you that? It was *your* decision. It was your life. Your children."

"That part you got right," responds Carolyn. "I'm glad we never had that discussion. It would have ended badly."

Carolyn explained that after her mother's deathbed diagnosis and finding out that other relatives of hers had died from the disease, she didn't want "any more surprises."

We were surprised, though, that her initial impulse had been just like Cheryl's—*not* to know. But as Carolyn moved into the last months of her second pregnancy, she had a change of heart.

Pregnant and worried, she remembers well the day her blood test came back: "I left work. I went to the office. I waddled in, took my envelope, went out to my car, took a deep breath, and opened it up."

The results? Negative. No FFI.

"That was a hallelujah moment," says Carolyn.

Carolyn has her hallelujah moment. Cheryl still has a mystery, preferring to continue living moment to moment.

IF THERE'S ANYTHING WE TOOK AWAY FROM OUR foray into the most mysterious diseases medicine offered us, it was a variation on what my mother, the anesthesiologist, often told me. "Honey," she would say when I complained of an ache or pain, "there are *billions* of processes going on in your body every second. Your sight, hearing, millions of red blood cells and platelets pumping through tens of thousands of tiny capillaries, internal gyroscopes, your liver filtering, your stomach acid dissolving, oxygen flying through your lungs' membranes, your brain firing electricity with every thought and memory. *Something's* going to go wrong every once in a while, and most of the time your body will fix it. When you think about it, it's a miracle that most of us make it through our lives *without* some sort of major disease. So take a hot bath, you'll live."

I have an even more profound gratitude toward my body now—its infinite complexity, and the fact that it keeps that complexity pretty much to itself. And all of us who've worked on *Medical Mysteries*—correspondents, writers, producers— have come away with an amazed admiration for the patients and doctors who help one another unravel these astonishing, challenging, perplexing diseases. Their courage is unbounded— as is our gratitude at being able to share their stories with you.

Acknowledgments

A talented, dedicated team did the research and production for the ABC television segments that gave rise to this book. It's an astonishingly collaborative process, and these incredibly hardworking professionals deserve our thanks. We've listed them in alphabetical order:

Joseph Angier, Rudy Bednar, Carol Berczuk, Nelli Black, Juju Chang, Kenneth Chu, Margaret Conley, Ramen Cromwell, Chris Cuomo, Andrea Fleischer, Mary Hanan, Catherine Harrington, Brad Hebert, Jacqueline Jaeger, Lynn Levy, Nian Liu, Allison Lynn, Kendra Macleod, Resa Matthews, Cynthia McFadden, David Muir, Sarah Namias, Jennifer Needleman, Lucy Orazem, John Quinones, Deborah Roberts, Megan Robertson, Jay Schadler, David Sloan, Trisha L. Sorrells, Maria Spinella, Bryan Taylor, Laura Viddy, Terry Wrong, Eleanor Yu.